The Effortless Sleep Companion

Also by Sasha Stephens

The Effortless Sleep Method

Coming in December 2013

Bedtime Stories for Insomniacs

The Effortless Sleep Companion

From chronic insomnia to the best sleep of your life

Sasha Stephens

Dark Moon Ltd

AUTHOR'S NOTE: The techniques, ideas, and opinions here are not intended as a substitute for proper medical advice. The information provided here is solely for informational purposes only. All information is generalised, presented for informational purposes only, not medical advice, and not to rely on this information as medical advice and to consult a qualified medical, dietary, fitness or other appropriate professional for their specific needs. This information has not been evaluated by any government agency and the information is not intended to 'diagnose, treat, cure or prevent any disease'. Any application of the techniques, ideas, and suggestions here are at the reader's sole discretion and risk. The author and the publisher expressly disclaim responsibility for any adverse effects arising from following this advice. While every effort has been made to ensure reliability and accuracy of the information within, all liability, negligence or otherwise, from any use, misuse or abuse of the operation of any methods, strategies, instructions or ideas contained in the material herein, is the sole responsibility of the reader.

Published by Dark Moon Ltd in 2013

The author and publisher of this material make no medical claims for its use. This material is not intended to treat, diagnose nor cure any illness. If you need medical attention, please consult your doctor.

Cover designer: Michael Warren
Copyeditor: Anna Carroll

A CIP catalogue record for this book
is available from the British Library.

First Edition

ISBN: 978-0-9571048-1-5

www.effortless-sleep.com
www.sashastephens.com

To Chipper.
Best friend, bedfellow, Siamese cat.

A word from your sleep angel

For you, dear insomniac, alone in the night, misunderstood, neglected and perhaps abused by the medical profession, for you, I am here ... now. I am not a doctor (thank goodness), nor do I pretend to be. But I can offer something different from every doctor you have come across ... *I know how it is to be you*, and I know how to make you better. Let me speak to you, perhaps like no one has ever spoken to you. Let me be your angel for the day. Let me help.

Contents

Why Should You Pay Any Attention to What I Have to Say?

So what makes me such an expert in sleep?

I was just an ordinary, moderately educated, moderate-class British woman, perfectly healthy and pretty happy, until insomnia struck. What followed was *15* years of appalling sleep problems.

I went on to suffer with acute, devastating insomnia, sometimes not sleeping at all for days. For 15 years I went through life in a waking nightmare of misery and exhaustion, with nothing ever helping, and no one ever understanding. During this time, I allowed insomnia to enter and affect every area of my life. At its height, I don't think I made a single decision without first assessing its possible effect on my sleep. Someone only had to say the word 'sleep', or 'insomnia', and my heart would leap, my ears would tune in and listen with fearful anticipation.

Good sleep became a mere memory for me and insomnia became my nemesis, my obsession … and my passion.

In 2005 a chance event enabled me to see the problem from an entirely new perspective. I had found a complete cure, *the* cure to my chronic insomnia, not in drugs or in external remedies, but by looking at myself, my behaviours, my thoughts and beliefs.

Following further research, I wrote my first book *The Effortless Sleep Method* in which I detailed the specific steps necessary to overcome chronic insomnia.

You can download the first chapter for free from www.effortless-sleep.com.

I was not prepared for the reaction to *The Effortless Sleep Method*. While I knew my insights would help some people, probably people like me, with problems just like mine, I had no idea I would be able to help people in all countries, of all ages, with all different sorts of insomnia. I did not expect to be able to help those with apparently 'physical' insomnia, those who had had a lifetime of suffering, sometimes for 30 or 40 years, those who had been diagnosed with chemical imbalances, psychological disorders, and even those with issues I *had not* experienced such as Restless Legs Syndrome, panic attacks and even nightmares. And I certainly was not prepared for the joyful, grateful letters of thanks I began to receive. People began to call me 'an angel', 'a Godsend'. It is a strange thing when someone tells you that you have 'given them their life back'. It is even stranger when it becomes an almost daily occurrence.

I maintain that only one who has suffered this affliction really has an insight into the problem – one who knows the intricacies of how it works, how it gets worse, and critically, what makes it better. I believe the chronic insomniac will never recover without this level of understanding. The chronic insomniac must come to realise that the 'cure' is entirely *and only* within their own power. If this sounds clichéd, it doesn't make it any less true.

The Effortless Sleep Method is the book I wanted someone to have written for me. During those 15 years I searched and scoured the world for a book like the one I have written. I searched for a person who really 'gets it', not some pompous doctor or dubious therapist, but someone who had been where I had been, someone who had been there, had those thoughts, *and who could tell me how to escape it.*

That person has come into your life. That person is me. *Please* don't think I am trying to be boastful here. If you think I sound arrogant, you have missed the point. I am not 'blowing my own trumpet' and I don't have a God complex. In fact, nothing could be further from the truth. I actually find self-congratulatory talk extremely uncomfortable, almost excruciating.

But I have to make you *believe* that I know what I'm talking about.

I tell you about people's gushing reactions just so that you can get an idea of what this method can do for you. My methods are controversial, and after suffering long-term insomnia, you may be bitter, sceptical, even cynical about the possibility of a mere book helping you, particularly if that book seems to contradict what doctors and other therapists have told you. The sooner I can break down that resistance the sooner you will begin to see results. And if boasting about how successful this method has been will serve to get you sleeping, then I'll do it, no matter how distasteful I find it.

My motivation for helping you is partly selfish. I had to go through agonies like yours for 15 years to get this knowledge. The only way I can make sense of what happened to my life during those terrible years is to turn this around: to use that experience to help people like me, like *you*, to be that person I had searched for. Without this, I would be left with a bitter resentment of my lost life. I *have* to help people like you now, *for my own sake.*

As my book became more successful, I didn't just receive letters of thanks. I also began to receive hundreds of letters, emails and blog comments with questions from people asking about their particular sleep problem. Each question received a full and personal reply and it would take me many hours almost every day to get through them all. When the questions started to become more numerous, and my time became scarcer, it was no longer physically possible to provide this service and I had to stop answering my own emails.[1] Instead, I began offering formal paid consultations. While answering the emails and carrying out the consultations, I noticed the same issues come up again and again. It was extremely rare for me to receive a completely new and unfamiliar question, and my answers, while all individual, tended to repeat quite similar advice. Before long, it became obvious that a second book would be the way to get *all* of this advice across to the maximum number of people for a fraction of the cost of a consultation.

For most, my first book is all it takes to cure a chronic problem. But for some, a little 'more' is needed – understanding doesn't quite 'bed in' from reading the book alone. So, for you 'tough nuts' I have created this second book, a more gritty, detailed, precisely targeted book, to answer all those little niggling questions you may still have, to deal with that obsessive thought, that pounding heart, that early waking, that waking with a start, and that difficult, oh-so-difficult-to-change negative belief 'I'm just a bad sleeper, there is something different here, nothing works for me, I'm getting worse ...'

This book contains answers to almost *every* question I have ever been asked and all the advice I have ever given up to this point

---

[1] Please don't email with your personal sleep questions. I am no longer able to answer the huge number I receive daily.

will be contained herein. If you have ever written to me, or have had a formal consultation with me, don't be surprised if some of this sounds familiar.

You should be prepared: I can be a little 'direct'. In the last book I didn't pull many punches. In this book I pull even fewer. I will not mollycoddle you, nor tell you what you want to hear. But I 'tell it like it is' and am absolutely honest in my advice. I tell it like it is because I want you to get over your sleep issues for ever. You see, I am not just here to help those who are already open to these ideas. I am also here for those who are very new to this sort of approach, to those who are convinced that their perfectly ordinary insomnia is a medical condition, for those who have never considered that thoughts and beliefs play a part in insomnia. I want to get through, not just to those who 'get it' straight away, but to those resistant, locked-down, know-best, heard-it-all-before types. Some people are very open to my ideas about sleep, but others are not. Some need a lot of convincing, and sometimes the only way to get through to the tough nuts is by not sugar-coating the message. The truth is I *particularly* want to help you tough nuts. I particularly want this because I know what it is like to be *you*. I know because, *'a resistant, locked-down, know-best, heard-it-all-before tough nut'* is exactly what I was for 15 years.

My intention is that after this book, there will be no more questions, no need to come to me for help. Having read this book, you should have all the understanding and all the knowledge you need to overcome *any* sleep problem.[2] I have done my utmost to make sure that your question, if you have one, has been answered by this book

---

[2] This does not include sleep apnoea or the 'parasomnias' such as sleepwalking or nightmares. If you suspect you have sleep apnoea, this is a potentially dangerous physical condition which needs to be treated by a doctor.

How to Read This Book

This book will help you to sleep better. I have worked hard to ensure the book you hold in your hands works as a standalone help for insomnia. Whether you have read *The Effortless Sleep Method* and still have questions, or are just starting out on your recovery and are entirely new to my writing, this book will give you new insights into your own problem and enough information to begin making the steps towards perfect, effortless sleep.

But in many respects, this book been written as a *companion* to the original Method. In what follows, I will not be covering the specifics of the Method itself. I highly recommend that you read this following or in conjunction with *The Effortless Sleep Method* in which full details of the essential steps are given.

This book is written in four stages. I call these *Understanding, Doing, Repairing* and *Being.* These are supposed to correspond loosely to the chronological progression of your recovery. As with all my books, you *must* read all sections in the order they are written. I put a lot of time and thought into the ordering of the information. Do not, under any circumstances, just skip to the bits you think look interesting. Even if it seems that a question posed does not apply to you, there may be something in my answer that does. Very often, understanding hinges on one little bit of information or inspiration. I wouldn't want you to miss that one little word or phrase that might make all the difference because it seems initially irrelevant. There is no one part which encompasses 'the cure', no key chapter, no single set of principles which will work alone to beat your insomnia. The book is written as a slow build, a steady teaching of the attitude and thinking required.

However, knowing what to do is only the beginning.

With a problem like insomnia, the intellectual part is *always* only a fraction of the battle. It is not by reading the book, but by experiencing the truth of it that you will overcome insomnia.

No matter how good an understanding you have, the only way my words will help you is if you *take action* on them, and start getting a feel for their truth. You need to experience the results of this advice, *not just to understand.*

Overcoming insomnia is largely not an intellectual process; it is an experiential process.

ॐ

Introduction
Why Me?

Do you remember life before insomnia? Do you remember when you were able to sleep anywhere, in any position, on the floor, in the moonlight, in a friend's bathtub? Remember when you were able to stay up all night, lie in all morning, drink double espressos after dinner and just … well … *live*, like a normal person? Remember when your every waking thought *wasn't* filled with thoughts about sleep? Remember when life was so free, so easy? Where did that life go? Where did that *person* go?

Perhaps you can't even remember. Perhaps your problem has been going on for so long that you can only look longingly to those around you to get an idea of how it would feel to be getting normal sleep. Perhaps you can only envy the lives and the sleep of others; the well-meaning but ignorant friends who think that taking 45 minutes to fall asleep constitutes a bad night. The ones who 'need two alarm clocks' to wake them, the ones who fall asleep in seconds, the ones who plan their carefree lives without the merest glimmer of a thought about sleep.

Whatever your story, you have probably, at some point, thought the following thought …

'Why me?'

Why *has* this happened to you? What disease or disorder do you have? What broke and how did it break? What's different about you?

If you are like most people, you probably just start off just missing a couple of nights. Perhaps you are ill or under stress, have a new baby, or a new job, a new relationship or a new home. Perhaps you are keeping weird sleeping hours, or doing shift work. You may be being disturbed by inconsiderate neighbours, or be sleeping in a strange bed. Or perhaps there is that one night where, for some inexplicable reason, you just can't sleep.

Usually, you are able to get back to normal sleep pretty quickly. But this time, things are different. This first sleepless night is followed by another, and another.

Your mother, friend or colleague perhaps suggests Valerian, passiflora or some other herbal remedy. But oddly, these things don't seem to do much good, despite coming so highly recommended. Why, you wonder, don't they work for you?

Within a few short days, the beginnings of fear set in. You find yourself worrying about whether you will sleep tonight, how much you *need* to sleep, how much you *must* sleep. You try to nap in the afternoon, but even that seems impossible. You lie down but sleep seems *miles* away. How can you be *this tired* and not be able to nap? You try to lie in at the weekend, to no avail.

Desperately aware of this need to sleep, you go to bed extra early one night, wide awake and in a panic. You try, and try, and *try* to relax, but you only become more and more awake. In fact, the more time you spend in bed trying to sleep, the more irritable you become. Perhaps tonight is your first ever night of no sleep whatsoever and you have to drag yourself through the next day, bemused and zombie-like, more tired than you ever thought possible.

Enough is enough. Only one thing for it: you do the sensible thing, the *recommended* thing, and go to your doctor. *That* will do it. The doctor will know what to do. He or she will almost certainly prescribe pills; probably Ambien (Zolpidem), Zimovane (Zopiclone) or perhaps Valium (Diazepam). These are proper, medically endorsed, clinically tested sleeping pills. *Thank goodness!* You know that sleeping pills are supposed to be bad for you, but let's face it: your problem is serious. If anyone needs them, *you* do! Tonight, you can put all this sorry business behind you. You'll get some lovely sleep and within no time you'll be back to normal.

The pills may work. But the sleep they give you doesn't seem to be as refreshing as you are used to getting. You may seem more anxious than usual, even a bit depressed. And after a short time, they seem to stop working quite so well, or they start to give you a nasty hangover. Sometimes they don't really work *and* give you a nasty hangover! And then that first terrible night comes along where you stay awake all night, right through the medication. And next morning you experience a whole different level of hell. This resultant hangover is worse than anything you have previously experienced. In fact, this is worse than *anything* the insomnia alone ever made you feel. These pills haven't made you *better*, they have made you *worse*.

Now what are you supposed to do?

You go back to the doctor's surgery to tell them of your strange and unexpected experience with the pills. The doctor reassures you; all you need to do is just increase your dosage, or try a different kind of pill. But the increased dosage doesn't work. The new prescription doesn't work … the increased dosage of the new prescription doesn't work!

You didn't expect *this*. Just what sort of insomnia do you have, that doesn't even respond to proper, medically prescribed sleeping pills? They have been researched and subjected to rigorous clinical trials. They are clearly working for other people. If they weren't working for people, doctors wouldn't prescribe them, would they?

You must have a really *severe* form of insomnia, a different, worse form than that of other people.

Perhaps you have some sort of imbalance in the brain, something hormonal, a lack of some vitamin or a food allergy, perhaps you have a genetic disposition to insomnia, perhaps your sleep mechanism has become damaged, perhaps a switch got turned on in your brain and you can't seem to turn it off.

Perhaps it's a control issue, perhaps it's an abandonment issue, perhaps you are scared of the dark, or afraid of sleep itself. Perhaps you are *sleep phobic.* Perhaps it's because you were bullied as a child, or had over-protective parents. Or perhaps it's because you can't stop your racing thoughts, your pounding heart, your sudden 'jumping' into wakefulness just as you are dropping off.

Or perhaps there is a genuine, physical, *real* reason for your insomnia. If *only* you could find the underlying *cause* of your insomnia, then perhaps you would know how to treat it.

In desperation, you turn to alternative treatments – herbs, CDs, relaxation techniques, and all sorts of strange therapies. Plenty of these help you in other ways, helping you relax or deal with troublesome issues. But they don't seem to touch the sleep. Some things work for a little while, but then stop working for no apparent reason. Some nights come along where *nothing* works.

And all the time, the fear is growing, developing, taking hold …

What went wrong?

What broke?

What's wrong with me?

What if I *never* get better?

What if I lose my job

What if I lose my husband/wife?

What if I can't look after my children?

What if I get *worse?*

What if I go mad?

What if I *die* of insomnia?

You start researching online, reading articles about insomnia, trying to find out all you can about your condition. You join some online support forums just in order to talk to someone, to feel less alone. And you discover, to your sick horror, that there are millions of people with insomnia all over the world, none of them getting any better, some of them suffering for *decades.* Hearing their stories only seems to add to your anxiety. Some of these people have suffered their entire lives, some of them have been hospitalised, had nervous breakdowns, spent time in mental institutions – is this what the future has in store for *you?*

Night-time has now become nothing to do with sleep. It is about panic, fear, phobia even. It is about loneliness, desperation, tears. You might even start getting the odd run of completely sleepless nights. Awake all night, followed by days of miserable, torturous hell.

Daytimes are spent in a confused combination of longing for bedtime and dreading it. You can't take any more. You *must* get some sleep. You need *help!*

Back to the doctor. Prescription pen out. Antidepressants this time. Insomnia and depression often go hand in hand, he or she tells you, so antidepressants are bound to help.

You might feel ambivalent about taking the antidepressants. Perhaps it just isn't path you ever wanted to go down. Perhaps it doesn't feel 'right'.

Or perhaps you are just relieved there is another approach, something, *anything*. Perhaps the antidepressant prescription comes as a blessed relief and you are *happy* to take them. Perhaps, right now, you are ready to try anything.

But you find, to your immense disappointment, that they don't help the insomnia at all. They don't even make you feel good. Or unbelievably, they make you feel *more* unhappy.

You may never have considered yourself depressed until the insomnia. You may be convinced that far from being caused *by* depression, insomnia has been *the cause* of your depression. In fact, it may feel like insomnia is the only thing standing between you and a great life.

But stand in the way it *does*. It stands in the way of fun, career advancement, relationships, light-heartedness, freedom, advancement, starting a family, self-development, spiritual growth ... no wonder people describe insomnia as a monster, as a curse.

Speaking to friends, no one seems to get it: 'If you're tired, why don't you just sleep?' they ask. Or they very helpfully say, 'You probably *do* sleep; you just can't remember it.'

No one gets it; not therapists, friends or relatives. In fact, not even the doctor seems to get it. Even the *sleep doctor* doesn't get it! What the hell is wrong with you?

Where did your life go?

CB

Stage One
Understanding
Will Set You Free ...

Let me get one thing straight.

Getting over your insomnia is not going to happen when someone invents a new cure, gadget or wonder drug. It's not going to happen when you discover the ideal, perfect therapist or relaxation technique. And surprisingly, it's not going to happen when you finally discover the deep-seated, hidden reason behind your insomnia or the original first cause.

And it is not going to happen just because you *do* what I *say*.

It's going to happen when you truly grasp the mechanics of insomnia, sleep and *your own problem*.

This requires understanding, true understanding. This book is my attempt to give you that level of understanding. By answering in great detail some of the most common questions asked of me, my hope is that the light bulb will go on in your insomniac mind. (Or rather, the light bulb will go off and let you sleep!)

In this book, it may seem that I repeat myself a lot. It's true; I do repeat myself. But I don't do this because I have run out of things to say. I do this intentionally. Repetition of these simple ideas will help you to remember, help you to understand. And, like many things, when it comes to insomnia, *understanding is power!*

A reviewer once said, 'Sasha doesn't just understand sleep; she understands the layered psychology of sleep.' Only by truly appreciating the layered psychology, the intricacies, the little nuances of your own problem, the way it works, the way you react, overreact and by seeing your own thoughts and behaviour for what they are, and the effect they have on you, can you be in a position of real power. A position that allows you to cope fully with whatever your insomnia throws at you. A position that means insomnia cannot frighten you any longer, a position which means you are totally able to cope with every set-back, every slip-up, and to use each little bit of progress as a rocket to success. A position which means you *know*, not just hope but *know*, that your battle with insomnia is over. You can only get to this position – not from sleeping pills, not from any external remedy, not even from my Sleep Tools or any relaxation technique I promote – you can only get to this position from complete *understanding*.

This will happen when you come to see all the things you *personally* have been doing to create and reinforce your insomnia, the mistakes you are making and the misunderstandings you have. It will happen when you finally 'get it' to the extent that you *stand up* to insomnia, no longer fear it, and watch it dissolve before your very eyes.

Your current position may feel like one of utter powerlessness. You may feel completely at the mercy of this problem. Right now, you are probably going to have trouble *believing* it, but perhaps you can *trust* that there is truth in what I am about to say.

You can turn this entire thing around.

You absolutely do have the power to take control of your sleeping patterns, your thoughts and even your life. I am not saying it will be easy, and you may have a lot of setbacks. But stay the course, give it time, and try to just trust that I do know what I am talking about. You *will* see results.

So first, just take a step back, a deep breath and resolve that you are going to stop running, stop panicking, stop letting this thing control you. You are going to commit to facing this, calmly examining your thoughts and following instructions. This may sound impossible right now because your mind is going to jump in and be all over this like a rash, and that's fine. All I am looking for is a *willingness*, an intention, if you like. Make a decision now, to take control of your sleep and your life. Just make that decision yourself, and I will show you how to do the rest.

Ready? Good. Now let's begin.

What Insomnia is Not

'My insomnia is different from and much worse than normal insomnia. Can you help people like me?'

The world of the insomniac is a lonely place. It seems that no one understands what you are going through, not therapists, not even doctors. Because sleeping pills and other remedies haven't helped, and because it seems no one suffers like you do, and no one seems to understand, it is natural that you begin to believe that there is something different, something broken, something 'not quite right' about you. Normal sleepers look astounded when they hear about your problem. 'How do you *cope*?' they say. 'I would just *die* if I slept as badly as you!'

It may surprise you to know that *most* insomniacs believe that there is something different about their insomnia that makes them different, more severe, or incurable.

But just think about this for a moment. There are at least six million insomnia sufferers in the UK alone. Now, if every one of these people is thinking their insomnia is different, this means there must be at least six million different types of insomnia out there just in this one little country, each one distinct from all the others.

How likely is that?

Let me just give you a selection of some of the things I once believed about my insomnia. At some point or other, I was convinced that:

1. My insomnia was worse than anyone else's.
2. My sleep mechanism was broken.
3. My insomnia was somehow 'different'.
4. My 'sleep switch' had got stuck in the wrong position.
5. I would never get better.

Here's the truth:

1. There were (and still are) millions of people with insomnia just as bad as mine (and yours).
2. There's no such thing as a sleep 'mechanism'.
3. My insomnia was just the same as any other old insomnia.
4. There's no such thing as a sleep switch.
5. I absolutely *did* get better.

One thing which contributes to this feeling of 'different-ness' is that unlike other ailments, which may fit into neat categories, insomnia doesn't seem to have clearly defined borders. It is a very 'fuzzy' concept. Some people can't fall asleep, some fall asleep easily but can't *stay* asleep, some sleep better away from home, some can never sleep away from home. Some have a problem with relaxation, some with a pounding heart or twitching limbs, others with racing thoughts or suddenly leaping into wakefulness just as they are about to drop off. Some never feel sleepy; some always feel tired no matter how much they sleep. Some find pills, potions, sleep aids, relaxation, or hypnosis helpful; some find none of these seems to work.

Sadly, the 'experts' usually do nothing to help you feel normal. I despair of hearing stories of sleep therapists and doctors suggesting wild and outlandish reasons for a person's insomnia. Or worse, experts often express disbelief, confusion or complete bewilderment, as if *yours* were the severest, most abnormal case of insomnia they had ever come across.

I know from bitter personal experience just how detrimental an effect these 'diagnoses' can have. I saw a top sleep therapist in London's prestigious Harley Street. This specialist came with a two-month waiting list and at a cost of thousands of pounds. He basically told me to practise Sleep Restriction and take drugs. When that didn't work he told me I need to 'just stop panicking'. His advice about how to do this? Relax more by petting my cat!

One of Britain's top hypnotherapists (also with offices in Harley Street) concluded that, as his therapy hadn't had helped, the only possible reason for my problem had to be a traumatic memory, which we needed to uncover over the course of many months. We never did uncover that traumatic memory.

I waited six months to see a National Health Service psychiatrist who seemed bemused by my story, as if it were the strangest tale he'd ever heard. He also offered drugs, which were refused, and then told me he basically couldn't help.

And, if the very best the country has to offer can't help us, then we imagine we must be *really broken, really severe ... incurable.*

We all think this. It doesn't make it true.

Yes, there are variations of insomnia. There are subtle differences between individual problems. But don't imagine for one second, just because pills don't work, doctors have given up on you and that nothing has worked for you so far, *that you are different.*

After reading this book, I hope that you will feel a lot more normal. You will find yourself in company with people *just like you.* Whatever your problem, the chances are I have probably seen it *and cured it.*

'But we aren't all exactly the same. Some of us turn into insomniacs, while others don't. So there is something different about us, isn't there?'

I have come to realise that there *is* one thing that sets insomniacs apart, possibly even the one thing which explains why some people develop chronic insomnia following a spell of mild sleeplessness, while others just go back to sleeping normally. But it is not what you would expect.

Let's have a little look at the anatomy and creation of a chronic problem. For most people, insomnia begins innocently enough – as a completely normal reaction to stress, irregular sleeping patterns, illness, medication or some other innocuous trigger. This sort of thing happens to millions of people every day, of every age, of every class, in every culture, all over the world. When left alone, this short-term trouble with sleeping usually rights itself with no outside assistance. The stress diminishes; the sleeping patterns normalise, and sleep returns.

But the *chronic insomniac* usually has a different story:

Inevitably, just a short while after the problem's onset, this person starts 'doing things', 'trying things', panicking and, quite often, taking pills. They then seek therapy, see umpteen doctors, discuss sleep with their friends, parents, colleagues, read up, research, stress, wonder, ruminate, analyse inside and out, go to pieces, and panic over something which doesn't faze a 'normal' sleeper. Sooner or later, fear of not sleeping sets in, this fear stops them sleeping which in turn feeds the fear of not sleeping, and they are off, set in a vicious circle of fear → insomnia → fear ... a fully fledged insomniac.

In other words, some people *overreact* to a bout of missed sleep. And I believe *it is this reaction alone* which is the defining characteristic of the chronic insomniac.

Notice that according to this version of events, whatever caused your first bout of sleeplessness in the first place is completely irrelevant. It is not the first cause, the underlying key issue, the physical condition, the trigger event, but what you did from that point on that turned it into the problem it is now. Chronic insomnia usually has little to do with physical causes or underlying trigger events. Chronic insomnia is largely a condition of *chronic over-attention to a problem.*

'So, is it fair to say that there is something about me, even if psychological, that makes me susceptible to insomnia?
Am I naturally just a bad sleeper?'

I actually do believe that there exist naturally weaker sleepers because I am the perfect example of this. I was always, and still am, a very *light* sleeper, meaning I am very easily wakened from sleep. I normally get up at least once a night to use the loo. I also find it almost impossible to nap, have *never* slept on a plane, and have almost always taken around an hour to fall asleep. So it's probably *true* that there are good and bad sleepers, in the sense that their sleep is *delicate.*

And then … there are those who panic and pay too much attention to a normal run of bad sleep.

And perhaps, when *both of these tendencies come together,* as they did with me (and maybe with you), then the really chronic insomniac is born.

THE EFFORTLESS SLEEP COMPANION | 25

'Aha! So I am different; I knew I was!'

What I have just said makes it sound like I am suggesting that there *is* something fundamentally 'different' about the chronic insomniac. I admit, insofar as this overreaction goes, there *is* something that sets the insomniac apart from normal sleepers. But it's nothing really to do with sleep, or the sleep response, or the sleep mechanism, or anything fixed in the brain. It is not a physical condition or deficiency.

Because this 'thing' that causes, creates and reinforces chronic insomnia is *perfectly changeable*. There is nothing fixed about this tendency to overreact and panic. I know, from personal experience, that delicate, bad sleepers *can become* good sleepers.

I don't know if you subscribe to my Bedtime Story emails. In July 2012 I wrote a bedtime story in which I wrote 'I have just woken from the best sleep of my life'. I was telling the truth. I had fallen asleep very quickly and slept right through the night, to wake up with a big smile on my face, a few minutes before my alarm. I can't put into words just how deep and delicious that sleep was. Since then, I have had many, many similar experiences. I am 44 years old and I am *still* getting better. And it's not just me. I regularly get letters from people in their 60s who have had a lifetime of sleep problems, reporting that they are sleeping better than they have ever done. I'm not saying this to rub your nose in the success of others, I'm doing it to try to prove to you that being a bad sleeper is not set in stone; a bad sleeper *can* become a really great sleeper.

And someday, I fully intend to be sleeping on plane journeys … someday.

*'But my insomnia IS different: I have an actual, medical
condition. How is it possible to help people like me?'*

I get many, many letters and emails from people who claim to
have a real, physical problem, chemical imbalance, or otherwise a
'biological' or 'medical' reason for their insomnia. Sometimes they
claim, 'I was damaged by surgery', 'have a neurological
condition', 'had a bad reaction to a drug', 'I have an idiopathic
syndrome'.

I have a real ambivalence when it comes to the value of diagnoses
such as these. On the one hand, the diagnosis gives you relief, that
you finally understand what the hell has gone wrong with your
body. It gives you understanding, vindication and a realisation
that you are not going mad, that there is something genuinely
wrong, something medical, something 'biological'.

But, 'idiopathic syndrome' or 'repetitive depressive syndrome' are
actually just clever-sounding ways of saying 'something weird
happened and we doctors can't explain it, so we'll give it a name
and it will sound like we still know what we are talking about.
And best of all, *it still sounds medical*, hence we are still in charge.'

However, it is for all these reasons that such an official-sounding,
'medical' diagnosis can also have a devastating effect on such
conditions that are exacerbated by negative thoughts and beliefs.
Insomnia is most definitely one of those conditions.

I now see people coming to me with all sorts of new psychological
'conditions' to explain their insomnia – Generalised Anxiety
Disorder (GAD), Repetitive Depression Disorder, Non-specific
Depressive Disorder, Adjustment Disorder, Maths Anxiety
Disorder (seriously!). And each time I hear this sort of 'diagnosis' I
want to scream. All these sorts of diagnoses do is to convince the
'patient' that they are suffering with a clearly defined, medical

condition. It cements, solidifies and makes their spate of insomnia utterly real. They 'have' something, a *real* condition, and *this* is why they can't sleep, *not* because they have simply got into an unhelpful thought pattern, nothing to do with their rotten sleep habits, but because they have something akin to a disease! And what do we do with diseases? Well, there are only two things: we cut people up or we give them drugs.

Of course many, many insomniacs begin their problem after an illness or after taking a particular medication. But very often the insomnia remains long after the illness has been completely overcome. The persistent belief that 'the insomnia is caused by the illness' means that these insomniacs tend to have a much harder time believing that there is *any* psychological aspect to their problem. It may even be that the 'physical' diagnosis of insomnia has a worse effect on the sleep than the initial adverse drug reaction or the illness itself. Because you have been given a 'real', 'medical', 'biological' reason for your insomnia, you obviously are going to have the classic insomniac belief that I talk about in my first book – 'my insomnia is different', more *real*, or at least 'more difficult to cure'.

This is not a crazy idea I have made up. Doctors are now well aware of the *nocebo effect*. This is the negative effect of a diagnosis or inactive treatment, the complete opposite of the *placebo* effect.

Let me digress with a little story from my own life. I think it would be appropriate to share this with you at this point. Years ago, before my insomnia started, I worked for a short time as a mortgage advisor. This job often involved my attending large meetings of hundreds of people, sitting listening to a speaker. Now, one day, right in the middle of a talk, I choked on a sip of Diet Coke. This set off an enormous coughing fit which lasted for ages. I ended up having to get up and leave the hall with hundreds of people looking at me choking and sputtering. It was very embarrassing. A couple of weeks later, I was again sitting in a large hall, listening to a different speaker, drinking another can of Diet Coke (I was convinced the caffeine helped me concentrate) when my mind wandered back to the previous coughing fit. Immediately, I began to feel a tickle in my throat. As I tried to suppress it the tickle grew worse and I felt the urge to cough. I coughed, once, but the tickle didn't go away. An enormous panic flooded over me as I realised that another coughing fit was imminent. Once again, I had to get up and leave, with everyone watching me. But this time it was even worse: the speaker, having remembered my last outburst, said over the PA system, 'Aren't you the girl who coughed last time?'

This incident signalled the beginning of a long and horribly embarrassing habit of coughing in meetings, cinemas and public places. Of course, I imagined it was the Diet Coke that had caused it, and I gave up not just Coke but coffee, tea and chocolate, started taking all manner of cough syrups and sucking lozenges (none of which made a blind bit of difference). Now it felt real, very real. I would start to feel a maddening tickle almost as soon as I sat down, and as I tried to suppress the tickle, the coughing would start. In fact, I could now kick off a coughing fit at *any* time, and I had an almost permanently sore throat.

This problem was *real*. In a sense, the problem *had* been caused, initially, by the Diet Coke. But the problem now was nothing to do with Coke or caffeine at all, but was all to do with my overreacting to a particular unpleasant situation.

Only looking back now can I appreciate that the coughing fit problem was just a rehearsal for my future insomnia problem. These days, I tend to believe that the mind, tension and anxiety can cause pretty much any physical symptom. I'm even starting to wonder how much serious illness is caused, or at least exacerbated, by our thoughts.

There was a time when it seemed I would *always* have some form of this behaviour happening in my life. Because as soon as the coughing stopped, I began to get tummy aches whenever I had anything important or fun to look forward to; and as soon as the tummy aches stopped, the anxiety headaches began, and as soon as the headaches stopped, the insomnia began. And ... the insomnia lasted 15 years.

Now, why am I telling you all this?

I want you to see that insomnia and my coughing problem have very strong parallels. In *The Effortless Sleep Method* I invented a mythical condition, 'solagaraphobia', which is the fear of being blinded by sunlight. I argued that by giving a name to a normal everyday occurrence (being momentarily startled by the sun) we could develop a more serious and permanent problem, *just from the diagnosis itself.*

Now, each of these serious problems (insomnia, habitual coughing, solagaraphobia) started after a particular event or situation – a period of stress, drinking Diet Coke, being blinded by sunlight, a medication, illness, or a poor routine. But in all these cases, there is no one, true, fundamental, physical, biological *reason* underlying any one of these problems. The initial causes are no longer even *relevant.* All that is left, in *all* of these cases, is the fear, the anxiety, and hence the 'reification' – making real – of a problem. I put it to you that with insomnia, the main reason for this 'condition' is *habit.* Insomnia is just a *bad habit.*

I'm next going to say something a little strange and not just a little controversial.

There is no such thing as insomnia.

What I mean by this is that insomniacs do not 'have' a condition which marks them out as incurable. They are not a different breed of person. They simply have some bad habits. Although I do talk about 'insomnia' and 'insomniacs' because it's difficult to make myself understood without them, I am seriously considering whether it's possible to eliminate these terms completely from my writing. Because, in a very REAL sense, you do *not* have insomnia; you are *not* an insomniac. This 'condition' does not exist in its own right. It's just a word we give to some nights where we didn't sleep very well.

> *'But I keep hearing that lack of sleep will affect my long-term health and I'll end up with a serious illness because of it. That sounds pretty real to me!'*

Many people become *terrified* they are threatening their health, even their very *lives* with sleep deprivation, having been told again and again that getting less than eight hours sleep means instant death or some other such nonsense. This type of scaremongering makes my blood boil. It is just this sort of horror story which can strike terror into the heart of the insomniac. Telling someone 'get some sleep or you'll die' is hardly conducive to good sleep. It's like telling a depressed person 'cheer up or you'll have a nervous breakdown!'

As far as I can see, there is very little evidence to support this. All the studies I have found were on those who were insomniacs but were also taking sleeping pills their entire life. I sometimes wonder if this is propaganda put about by drug companies, to try to lure desperate insomniacs into eight hours of drugged sleep. I can direct you to another study done by arch sleeping pill opponent, Dr Daniel Kripke,[3] which concludes the *exact opposite!* He found that those who sleep around six hours *live longer!*

Please remember that I suffered for 15 years with very little sleep, sometimes going days and days without any sleep at all. And if my own case is anything to go by, 15 years of near-madness over insomnia doesn't seem to have done me any physical or psychological harm at all. I feel saner and healthier than I ever have done and I have never had any type of serious illness (touch wood!). I know I'm only one case, but I am the healthiest person I know. I almost never go to the doctor and haven't seen a specialist or consultant of any description since the psychiatrist I mention in the book. That was over 20 years ago.

'But what about vitamin deficiencies, hormone levels, food intolerances, traumatic events in one's past? Are you suggesting that these things don't affect sleep?'

Of course they can affect sleep. But we aren't talking about odd days or times in our life when we just don't seem to be sleeping too well. We are talking about the type of long-term crippling insomnia which takes over a person's entire life. A traumatic event or hormonal fluctuations may give us the odd bad stretch of sleep, or be the initial cause of a bout of sleeplessness. But once chronic insomnia bites, that event or trigger becomes irrelevant. It is not the event, the deficiency or the hormones that cause chronic insomnia; it is *what you are doing now.*

---

[3] Kripke, D. F., Garfinkel, L., Winguard, D. L., Klauber, M. R. and Marler, M.R. (2002) Mortality associated with sleep duration and insomnia. *Arch Gen Psychiatry*, 59, 131–136.

I certainly accept that vitamin deficiencies and diet can play a part in quality of sleep. (You can't go wrong with a good vitamin B complex.) I also know that my eating too much sugar at night results in a kind of hangover, that I sleep a bit better in the first half of my menstrual cycle to the second, and that my overall mood is improved by avoiding getting drunk. But I don't believe that there has ever been a case of chronic insomnia which has been cured by cutting out wheat or taking vitamin B. Sorting out your diet, reducing alcohol, taking vitamins, etc. will all serve to improve general health and can make the quality of your sleep a bit better. But just because this is true, does not make any of these things a cure for chronic insomnia.

'But surely you must acknowledge the possibility that I have an underlying physical ailment?'

I'm not saying it's impossible that there is a physical reason for your insomnia. It would be ridiculous, unfair and downright ignorant of me to suggest such a thing. It could well be the case that your insomnia is caused by a physical problem or that a drug you are taking is having an unwanted effect. All I am saying is that there is probably no way for you tell how much of an effect (if any) the physical problem is really having on your sleep and how much of it (if any) is being caused by negative thinking and poor expectation.

Consider how incredibly sensitive sleep is to suggestion; just the thought of not being able to sleep is strong enough to cause a sleepless night. In light of this it would be *incredible* if worry about the physical problem or the diagnosis itself did *not* having a detrimental effect on sleep. You don't know that what you have is not just an ordinary case of insomnia alongside a physical ailment.

Over the years, I have been contacted by many people who claim to have genuine, physical reasons for their insomnia. With *very* few exceptions, I have still yet to be convinced by any insomniac who claims their problem is physical. This is not because I am stubborn or ignorant, or because I'm down on the medical establishment (which I am, coincidentally). It's because:

1. The insomnia of those who believe their insomnia is physical exhibits exactly the same characteristics as the insomnia of those who don't.

2. I often see these same people with an apparently physical diagnosis go on to overcome their problems using purely 'psychological' and behavioural methods.

In fact, in terms of recovery, I have not noticed any major difference between the success of those with a 'physical' condition, and those who are sure their problem is purely psychological. In my experience, there is no correlation at all between lack of success and claims of a physical cause for insomnia.

So, how do you determine whether your condition is genuinely based on a physical ailment? Well, that's easy. Ask yourself the following questions:

- Do you fear not sleeping?
- Do you fall asleep quite easily, only to awake a few hours later, unable to get back to sleep?
- Do you take naps, lie in bed at weekends or have very irregular sleeping times?
- Do you sleep badly before important events?
- Do you sleep worse when under stress?
- Do you have low expectations of sleeping?

- Does your insomnia get better or worse on holiday?
- Do you sleep better on weekends or when you don't have to get up for work?
- Are you constantly trying new things to cure your insomnia?
- Do you sleep better or worse in a strange bed?
- Does fear of not sleeping sometimes keep you awake?
- Do you get more and more anxious as bedtime arrives?
- Do you find yourself falling asleep, only to awaken with a jolt?
- Do you find yourself waking up in the night in a panic?
- Do thoughts about insomnia occupy a large part of your day?

And, most importantly, have you noticed *any* connection between worry, fear or environment and lack of sleep, *even if* you are *sure* there is an underlying biological reason for the sleeplessness?

If you have answered 'yes' to even *one* of these questions: good! *Excellent*, in fact. Because these are not indicators of a biological condition; these are very much indicators of a psychological and/or behavioural condition, just like every other 'normal' insomniac. If the answer to even *one* of these questions is yes, then at least *part* of your problem is not physical. End of story.

Now, don't jump to defend yourself and your condition, because this is *good news*. This means I can help you; this means you can recover, just like any ordinary insomniac. Now, it's perfectly possible that there is a physical condition which makes sleep much harder to come by. But by answering 'yes' to more than a couple of these questions you tell me that the psychological and behavioural side is probably a much greater problem. Sort out the sleep behaviour and the psychological side of things and the physical problem could become nothing more than an annoying niggle for your sleep.

But moreover, if you *don't* sort out these other aspects, then even if you *cured* the physical issue completely, the chances are the insomnia will remain a problem long after that initial physical cause has been cured and forgotten about.

I read a Facebook comment recently. The commentator had responded to a post from a woman who had found meditation had cured her insomnia. The comment was very dismissive, saying something along the lines of 'If she managed to cure insomnia with meditation then she can't really have had proper insomnia in the first place.' So wedded was this man to the idea that his insomnia was real, was medical, was incurable, that he could not allow the possibility that someone else had overcome it so easily. Don't be one of these people. Don't choose to hang onto your insomnia rather than consider a new idea.

Now, some of you will still want to fight me on this. Some of you will react with anger, feeling patronised and even insulted. But ask yourself this: what are you defending? Why is it so important that you make me wrong? Wouldn't it be better *for you* if I were right? But hey, it's your life. You can go on believing there is a physical cause for your insomnia, and wait until a medical cure comes along, all the while acting as guinea pig for every new vile and dangerous sleeping pill which comes out of the pharmaceutical companies' labs, *or* you can decide now that it's at least as much a psychological issue as it is a physical issue and let me help you. The worst that can happen is nothing at all, I will be wrong and all you have wasted is a few pounds on a book. If you go down the medical route, the worst that can happen is … well, terrible, quite frankly.

Don't be one of those who try to prove me wrong.

'I think you are wrong to blame the victim when actually this is the responsibility of doctors. More should be done by doctors to find a proper medical cure. Just because there isn't a cure yet doesn't mean there never will be.'

Please believe that I'm not trying to bully you into believing me just to win the argument; really I'm not. I want you to see the immense danger in the belief that insomnia is based on a physical condition. I say this because, unlike most doctors, *unlike most sleep specialists*, I actually have experience of *curing* (not drugging) thousands and thousands of chronic insomniacs. I only say these things in an attempt to help you, honestly. So please, whenever you hear me say something you don't agree with, understand that I say such things, not to prove any points, but only to help you.

Having suffered myself for 15 years, what reason would I have for blaming the victim? What possible motivation would I have for doing that? To let myself off the hook? Because I don't have any other answers? I don't need to do any of these things. I don't have any obligation to come up with any answer whatsoever. I was a victim too, once, remember?

The very worst problem with not accepting my way of seeing things is that it is actually completely disempowering. It's *only* by taking responsibility (which is completely different from 'accepting blame') that you have *any* hope of getting relief, of doing anything about this. I say that your recovery is your own responsibility, not because I have no other answers, but *because it's true*. And, moreover, if I'm wrong and it's *not* true, *then you are left powerless*.

Are you going to sit around and wait for doctors and drug companies (who have been less than no help so far) to trial drug after drug on the victims of this horrible problem? Or are you going to do whatever you can to take control of your own life?

While you continue to believe that medicine will one day be the answer, you are basically at the mercy of the doctors. Or, more accurately, at the mercy of the drug companies (which is about the worst possible place on earth to position yourself.) If you really believe that this is a physical problem, it means you are crippled. You are stuck. You are powerless. You will remain broken, until some unknown date when doctors can get to you.

So, isn't it *great news* that I *don't* believe it's a physical problem? Isn't it *great news* that I actually have *an answer*, because right now, the doctors have no answers, absolutely none.

So, can I make a suggestion? Treat your insomnia with my methods while you are waiting for the physical cure to come along.

'But what about insomnia due to terrible pain or a stimulant drug, steroids, for example.'

Yes, okay, I would agree that there is probably a lot less of a psychological aspect in this situation. But then, is this sort of sleeplessness really insomnia at all? If I stand in your room and poke you with a stick all night, is that insomnia? If I shout 'Wake up!' in your ear every half hour, is that insomnia? If you have a completely separate condition that makes it difficult to sleep, like terrible pain, then *that* is surely the thing that needs your attention? If you can't sleep because you have terrible pain, get a book on terrible pain. Trying to treat this sort of sleeplessness as normal insomnia is like looking for effective pain relief when you have a knife stuck in your chest, or trying to sort out your posture when you have a broken back.

'But what about insomnia due to stress? You can't tell me that that is anything to do with sleep habits and poor thinking.'

I will have a lot to say later on the subject of stress, anxiety and physical tension. Certainly, stress is probably the most common initial cause of a bad bout of sleep. When stressed and very anxious, sleep can be near-impossible to find.

However, sleep very often remains bad once the stressful event or situation has passed. Any insomnia left behind is then down to poor belief, low expectation and less-than-ideal sleep habits. But complicating the issue is the fact that very often the stress or anxiety is *about* insomnia and thus is absolutely to do with poor thinking. Even when stress remains high, just by working on negative thinking and tightening up sleep hygiene, it is still often possible to make sleep a lot easier to come by.

'What about genetic insomnia? My mum is a bad sleeper, and so was my grandma. My sister doesn't sleep too well either. How do you explain all that unless insomnia is hereditary?'

Do I believe that insomnia can be genetic? No, not in the slightest. However, if you ask whether it runs in families, then my answer is yes! But insomnia runs in families in the same way that smoking runs in families. These things are not genetically encoded; they are *taught.* They are *learned.* So don't get hung up on the idea that other family members suffer with insomnia. This is no more than a reaction to negative messages about sleep.

'I hear what you are saying, but I do have one particular issue which I am sure is the reason for my insomnia. I know that if only I could get over this particular issue I could sleep fine.'

Very often, the insomniac focuses acutely on one particular aspect of the problem which they believe to be the absolute crux, the key to curing their insomnia. This may be a particular mind or relaxation state, one particular belief or a physical issue.

- 'I can't stop this fuzzy/achy/wobbly/weird feeling; if I could, I know I could sleep.'

- 'I am almost falling asleep and then something wakes me with a start. I just need to find out what that thing is that wakes me, then I'll be able to sleep.'

- 'I am sabotaging or punishing myself. I need to find out why that is before I can sleep.'

- 'I used to read to help me sleep. Now it wakes me up. I must find out why I can't sleep after reading. Then I'll be able to sleep.'

- 'I get this strange situation where I am really relaxed and almost fall asleep but never quite lose consciousness. That is what I need your help with.'

- 'I have control issues. I need to learn to relinquish control before I can sleep.'

Do you feel there is one specific reason for your insomnia, or one 'thing' you need to beat, learn or deal with? Do you visit doctors, therapists just trying to sort out this *one* issue? Did you skim through this book, just looking for reference to 'your' particular issue? (This is the reason I refuse to add an index!)

You may feel that because your problem involves some *particular* circumstance, the usual advice doesn't apply. Before even finishing (or even starting) the book, some of you will write to me with questions. Such questions might be:

- 'My problem is I never feel sleepy. Have you heard of this before?'

- 'My mind is always full of racing thoughts. How can I stop them?'

- 'My insomnia started after pregnancy/illness/trauma. What is your specific advice for someone like me?'

- 'I sleep fine for a few days and then can't sleep for no reason at all. Why do I always relapse like this?'

- 'I can't control my thoughts at all. What is wrong with me?'

- 'My insomnia is stress-related. Do you address this?'

- 'My insomnia is not stress-related. Do you cover this in your book?' and so on and so on.

Some people also 'diagnose' themselves with some particular special form of insomnia. For example, 'I have genetic insomnia', 'I have seasonal insomnia', 'I have psychophysiological insomnia', 'I have exercise-induced insomnia', 'I have depression-induced insomnia', 'I have insomnia-induced depression.' Sometimes they can write to me quite indignantly to inform me that their particular form of insomnia is *not* mentioned in my book!

Before you tell me that you have a special kind of insomnia, that your problem is different, or that your sleep mechanism is broken, *stop*. At some point, I thought all of these things. It may surprise you to know that pretty much everyone with a chronic problem thinks one or other of these things. It may also surprise you to know that almost invariably, none of them is ever true. These problems we think are the absolute crux of our problem turn out to be utterly irrelevant.

I speak often about the danger of looking for the root cause of your insomnia. Do this, and the mind will just run riot, making up theories, then arguing with those theories, twisting itself in knots trying to make sense of things. When in fact is there usually *is* no sense to be made regarding these things.

1. First of all: All this focusing on one specific aspect creates a nice strong point to which to anchor the obsession! 'Aha!' thinks the insomniac, 'It's all about *this*! Now, all I need to do is work out how to conquer *this*.' But trying to stop doing *this* is a little like trying not to think of a white bear. An obsession requires attention to keep it locked in, and this sort of attention is ideal for that purpose.

2. And secondly, if the sufferer does overcome this *key thing* there is always another just waiting to jump into the prime spot. Because this 'one key thing' never was what was causing the insomnia in the first place.

3. Forget about the 'one key thing' and there will cease to be 'one key thing' at all!

There is a strange phenomenon that happens sometimes when people write to me with a very desperate and specific question. I sometimes get people frantic for the answer to one nagging, crucial question they have. They sometimes offer me large sums of money if I can answer this *one* question, help them with this *one* thing which they *know* is the key to overcoming their problem.

Do you know what I do in these cases? I ignore them. That's right, I ignore them, for at least a week or two, telling them I don't have time to answer right now.

Then I come back a fortnight later to ask them how they are doing. *In almost all cases*, they have almost forgotten about the crucial issue that was bothering them! It may well be that in a few weeks or months you won't even *remember* this vital, crucial question. It simply won't be relevant any more. By focusing so intently on this sort of detail, an intelligent person is always going to find ways to pick holes, find exceptions, and come up with new ideas, new theories, *new problems*. Instead of trying to sort out particular details, we need to undermine the whole structure, shake it loose so that new symptoms or specific problems can no longer jump up and sabotage us.

> *'But if I find the underlying cause, or the trigger event, surely the problem will disappear. The internet is full of suggestions that you must find the thing that is causing your insomnia. Otherwise, what is the point of having years of therapy?'*

Is that last question rhetorical? I hope so. Because as far as I'm concerned there is no point in finding the one trigger event or deep-seated cause, and even less point in having years of analytic therapy! And if you start believing everything you read on the internet you will be in seven shades of trouble. In almost all cases there is *no* point in looking for a key cause for your insomnia.

I spent *years* in therapy trying to find out the key, trigger cause for my insomnia. Most therapists seemed to latch onto the early death of my father, suggest that it was an unconscious fear of death that was keeping me awake, or a fear of being abandoned if I let my guard down. One suggested that I had a control disorder which was causing my body to fight my mind, another that this was a form of self-sabotage – that I felt I didn't *deserve* to sleep. What utter nonsense!

I remember when I was convinced that this 'self-sabotage' diagnosis was the right one. I spent years and thousands of pounds inquiring into, analysing, therapising, treating my self-sabotage mechanism.

I also remember when I was convinced that my insomnia was a control issue. I was (and still am) a bit of a control freak. I spent years and thousands of pounds inquiring into, analysing, therapising, treating my control issue.

But when I had dealt with that issue, I remember instead thinking it was a fear issue, a fear of sleep, a sleep phobia. I spent years and thousands of pounds inquiring into, analysing, therapising ...

But the weird thing was, immediately that I had stopped theorising that fear of sleep was behind my insomnia, something else immediately jumped into the spot, to become the new object of my obsession. Some of these new candidates included:

- Focusing on the physical way I felt in the daytime – was I tired, were my eyes sore, was I relaxed, was my heart beating too fast?
- Diet. Lack of vitamin B, vitamin C, omegas 3 and 6, wheat intolerance.
- Another was overcoming this 'jump' into consciousness that would happen whenever I started to fall asleep – was it fear, control, excitement?
- And one thing which took up *years* of my focus was an obsession with trying to find the ideal sleeping position.

This last one stemmed from the knowledge that my insomnia appeared to start at a time in my life when I had suddenly started sleeping on my back, after 23 years of sleeping on my side. So sleeping position *had* to be relevant, didn't it?

(By the way, I never did go back to sleeping on my side. I still sleep on my back, wonderfully, and usually with a cat curled up in one armpit.)

Just to prove a point, here are some candidates for the underlying key reason or trigger for your insomnia:

- Your circadian rhythms are messed up.
- Not sleeping is hereditary in your family.
- Your ancestors were night-time hunters, and did most of their sleeping in the day.
- You have a deficiency of vitamin A, B, C, D, E, K, iron, calcium, potassium, oestrogen, progesterone, or testosterone.
- You have a wheat intolerance, dairy intolerance, sugar intolerance or some other intolerance.
- Your neuro-receptors have been damaged by drugs (this is a popular one).
- Your cortisol levels are too high/adrenals are burned out.
- God is testing you.
- God is punishing you.
- You have a control issue
- In a previous life you died in your sleep and now you are afraid to sleep.
- Someone once called you 'lazy' for sleeping too long and now you feel too guilty to sleep.
- You once woke up at work with everyone laughing at you for sleeping at your desk and now you feel too ashamed to sleep.

Take your pick.

Any one is as good or bad as the others. Now, I am not saying that none of these could be correct. Any one of all or any of these theories *could* in fact be true. The reason I reject them all is that there is absolutely no way for you definitively ever to find out!

> *'But just because we can't discover a hidden cause,*
> *doesn't mean there isn't one.'*

True. But what good does this do you? What good can it possibly do you to believe that there is a mystery, hidden cause which is impossible to discover? You might as well blame your insomnia on the pixies.

The upshot of this entire section is this: No matter what you believe to be the underlying cause of your insomnia, I ask that you allow yourself to be open, at least to the possibility, that chronic, long-term insomnia is largely a bad habit.

CB

Stage Two
Doing
Something about It

'Okay, I believe you. Now just tell me how to sleep.'

Many of us have some experience of overcoming a bad habit, perhaps smoking, drinking, overeating, too much coffee or chocolate, nail biting or thumb sucking. Attempting to break these types of habits always involves our stopping *doing* something. Now, this process may be very difficult, but with enough will-power, determination and strength of character, it is at least *possible* for a person even to give up a drug like heroin. This means that such habits are (at least in principle) completely under our control. Most of us try to use force, might or will to overcome the insomnia habit. But poor sleep is not like a heroin or nicotine addiction. While insomnia almost always involves bad habits, sleeping is not something we actively *do*. It is not something that can be forced, not something we can use brute, sheer will-power to overcome. We can hardly force ourselves to stop being awake! On the contrary, the greater the will, the stronger the character and the harder the attempt to sleep, *the more sleep eludes us.*

When trying to overcome insomnia, you may be tempted to focus intently on affecting and controlling the sleep itself, the falling asleep process, and the quality and duration of sleep. Thus you are concerned with what goes on in bed ... as you get in, as you get drowsy, the thoughts you have, the feelings you have as you fall asleep, or as you *try* to fall asleep. The level of consciousness, those sudden jerks awake as you become drowsy. You may become acutely aware of falling asleep itself, and try somehow to influence it. You may take a pill to 'make' you sleep. You may use all manner of sleep aids; you may even try bigger and more elaborate combinations of sleep aids and pills, as if by taking more, you can force yourself to unconsciousness.

Critically, you are probably particularly concerned with *doing* something on those nights *when you can't sleep.* I was always looking for something to *do*, to make me fall asleep on those nights when sleep eluded me – recordings, magnets, breathing and focusing techniques, having a whole armoury in place ready, in case tonight turned out to be a 'bad night'. Thus I was always focused intently on sorting out those bad nights if and when they occurred. After all, I reasoned, if I managed to sleep on those really *bad* nights, the good nights would take care of themselves. Thus, I spent most of my time as an insomniac focusing on *doing* as much as I possibly could *on* those bad nights.

As it turned out, this was all wrong. I didn't realise at the time that each bad night was the almost inevitable *end result* of a much more involved problem. Good or bad sleep is the inevitable result of a much longer chain of events. By the time a night came along 'when I couldn't sleep', it was usually too late. The damage was done. Once I had worked myself into an anxious, nervous state, there was usually *nothing* I could *do* to *make* myself sleep.

The changes we need to make are less to do with sleep *per se* than they are to do with the thoughts and behaviours surrounding sleep, those things that *lead* to sleep (or lack of it). Rather than focusing on the bad night itself, we actually need to be concerned with everything that has led up to it. Indeed, waiting until bedtime generally is the wrong approach. It is far, far better to work on getting the conditions right *before* bedtime comes. In many cases, bedtime activities are the least of what need our attention.

> *Beating insomnia is probably less than 10 per cent*
> *about what we do in bed.*

Instead, we must take a more 'holistic' attitude to insomnia. The habits we need to work on permeate our entire life; they are all those other things we do in our everyday lives which affect sleep. This means stopping doing those things which worsen our sleep and increasing those things which promote good sleep. We need to work on making things easy for sleep to slip back into your life. Not by trying to force it, or *make* it happen, not by drugging you, not by attaching you to magnets or by wearing special hats, but by *allowing* sleep. If we end up with very much still to 'do' at bedtime, that something will almost inevitably interfere with the falling asleep process. This is why many so people find bedtime relaxation techniques, CDs and mp3s actually wake them up. Ideally, we want there to be very little left to do once in bed. Good sleep is something that will generally occur naturally and effortlessly when the circumstances are right.

What so many insomniacs fail to realise is that sleep is never something they can *make happen*. So this book (like all my books) is not about giving you one word, technique, or bit of information or knowledge which will *make* you sleep; that isn't actually possible. I'm simply showing you how to go about instilling the good habits of thinking and behaviour that will *allow* sleep: real sleep, natural, non-drugged, effortless, *inevitable* sleep. Rather than trying to do something in bed 'when we can't sleep' we need instead to work on making the circumstances as conducive as possible *before* we get anywhere near the bed. Rather than fixing the bad nights, we need to prevent those nights from happening in the first place. And, I have discovered that the most conducive sleep conditions will always involve the following three factors.

The Tea Recipe for Sleep-Conducive Conditions

We Brits do love our tea. But the usual tea we serve with milk and biscuits is not a helpful aid to sleep, particularly when strong, and particularly when drunk at night. However, the sort of TEA I'm talking about is really, really good for sleep, especially when made properly. To get your sleeping back on track, and instil good habits in place of the bad ones, we need to attend to one, two or usually all three of the following.

T IREDNESS (specifically concerning actual sleepiness rather than daytime fatigue and exhaustion)

E XPECTATION (includes belief, thinking and association of bed and sleep)

A NXIETY (includes worry, stress, and physical tension)

Every promise and all of the advice I give in *The Effortless Sleep Method* can be boiled down to addressing one, two or all three of these three areas. When all three aspects are at the optimum level, sleep will occur naturally, without any need for external aids, pills or even techniques. But when one or more of these is widely off the mark (for example, if *anxiety* is too high or *tiredness* or *expectation* is too low) sleep will be hard to come by no matter what we do to help.

> *'It's ridiculous to suggest I work on my tiredness.*
> *Of course I'm tired. I'm bloody exhausted!'*

By 'tiredness' I don't just mean the ever-present feeling of anxious exhaustion which relentlessly permeates your life. I am talking about actual *sleepiness*, the feeling of being able to fall asleep at any moment. To illustrate the difference, think of the infuriating experience of being utterly shattered, but completely unable to nap. This happens because you are tired, exhausted even, but not *sleepy*. How is this possible? When someone helpfully suggests, 'If you're tired, why don't you just sleep', what is it that they don't understand? Why *can't* you sleep if you are so tired?

The reason is no matter how tired we are, if *anxiety* is too high (for example you are worried and tense), and/or *expectation* is too low (for example, when you try to take a nap at the 'wrong' time) you will be very tired without feeling remotely sleepy.

When the problem is new, a common reaction is to go to bed 'nice and early' or to try to take naps in the afternoon. This 'going to bed at the wrong time' when you are not actually feeling sleepy is a great contributor to the severity of an early problem.

Just by slightly increasing the tiredness levels, we can sometimes 'override' low to moderate levels of *anxiety* and poor *expectation* and allow sleep to happen simply with this one action. Increasing *tiredness* is the principle on which Sleep Restriction Therapy is supposed to help. Sleep Restriction involves drastically reducing the time you spend in bed, sometimes to as little as four or five hours. The idea is that by making you *so* tired, you sleep no matter how high your anxiety, or how low your expectation. It doesn't always work, as you may have discovered. Sleep Restriction is also *difficult* and can be very, very unpleasant.

I do recommend you increase your tiredness by cutting the time you spend in bed, especially if you are in the early stages of overcoming insomnia. But by attending to *anxiety* and *expectation* at the same time, the harsh, restrictive regime of Sleep Restriction Therapy is not necessary. As long as we attend to these other two aspects, cutting back your time in bed by ½ hour to an hour is usually all the restriction you need to improve your sleep.

However, if anxiety is very high, increasing *tiredness* slightly won't help. When we are *really* tense and anxious sleep becomes almost impossible even if on a strict Sleep Restriction plan. When we are very anxious, our heart beats faster, our adrenaline flows more and our minds are active. Our body goes into fight or flight mode and so keeps us awake to deal with danger. *Anxiety* (and associated physical tension) is often what keeps us awake for hours; it is what makes us feel physically stiff and uncomfortable when we get up after a bad night.

Even quite low levels of anxiety and tension will also affect your sleep cycle. A normal healthy sleep cycle is made up of just the right amounts of the three main types of sleep: Stage 1 sleep, deep Delta sleep and REM sleep. When very tense or anxious, this often leads to your getting large amounts of light Stage 1 sleep, and not much else. And if you're not also getting decent amounts of REM and deep Delta sleep, you aren't going to feel good in the morning, no matter how much light Stage 1 sleep you get. Deep dreamless Delta sleep is the most refreshing and even just a couple of hours of this delicious type of sleep can leave you feeling better than any number of hours of light Stage 1 sleep.

Anxiety caused by a particular stressful event or circumstance is responsible for many cases of sleep-maintenance insomnia. This is when you find it relatively easy to drop off, only to wake a couple of hours later unable to get back to sleep. If you started suffering sleep-maintenance insomnia at the same time as the appearance of a particular or new stress in your life, attending to your anxiety levels with yoga, exercise or meditation may well be all you need to improve things.

Most sleep medicines, including prescribed medication and over-the-counter remedies, are created to reduce anxiety and physical tension, to the extent that they cause the opposite state in us – *drowsiness*. For those who don't have a history of insomnia, these remedies can work well. If your only problem is that you are a little tense sometimes, a simple chemical relaxant will be all you need to drop off.

But without working to reduce the *underlying* stress, tension or anxiety, these drug remedies are only ever a temporary fix. They simply dull the pain of anxiety, not removing it permanently. Sometimes (particularly when expectation of a good night's sleep becomes almost zero), they don't even dull the anxiety. In these cases, the taking of a sleeping pill can actually *cause* anxiety. The person may try, sometimes unconsciously, to fight the effect of the drug. Fears about next-day hangover, or guilt over having succumbed to medication, can also lead to massively *increased* anxiety and even panic.

The first step in combatting insomnia is always to attend to these two aspects – *anxiety* and *tiredness*. Get these things right first. *This may be all you need* to overcome insomnia, particularly if your problem is recent. So the first two steps, *for everyone*, are as follows:

1. Do some serious de-stressing activities to reduce anxiety.
2. Create ideal tiredness levels by instilling good *sleep hygiene.*

Sleep hygiene is a set of 'going-to-bed habits' designed to create the ideal conditions for sleep. My first book, *The Effortless Sleep Method,* goes into a lot more detail regarding *sleep hygiene* – the mechanics behind good sleep habits and the reasons why these are so essential to beating insomnia. You will learn some of these essential sleep hygiene rules later in this section.

Sleep hygiene will ensure you have optimal *tiredness* levels.

Introducing a regular relaxation routine into your life will deal with any underlying tension or *anxiety*. (More on this later.)

If you still see no real improvement once these first two aspects have been taken care of, then there can only be one thing left which needs attention – *expectation.*

You may already have worked hard on your tiredness with good sleep hygiene. You may have a comprehensive set of de-stressing activities in place to deal with anxiety. But if your thoughts remain full of fear and negativity, expectation will stay low and insomnia will continue to plague you. Low expectation is so powerful it can override everything else, keeping you awake even when your tiredness and anxiety levels are good. When insomnia bites, low expectations of sleeping set in quickly. Even those whose problem is of short duration can develop really poor expectation, and even fear.

Expectation is fed by our very thoughts, often every moment of the day, and this makes it a particularly tricky customer. If you bought the first book, this will be the reason you bought the second. This is the reason most of you are here. This is the thing that trips up most people, and is the hardest thing to change.

Medication (and sleep aids) *can* increase expectation in some circumstances. Because you believe and trust absolutely that the drug will work, it does. This is most apparent in those people whose expectation and trust in the drug are so strong, they find the tiniest crumb of a pill will often put them to sleep, even on a bad night. The idea behind the prescription of a short course of sleeping pills is to break the insomnia habit by normalising sleep patterns, and so instilling a *new* habit. In theory, this sounds reasonable. But let's look at the kind of expectation that medication promotes. The expectation is not in one's own ability to sleep, not in the idea that insomnia is being overcome. It is rather expectation and trust in an external pill. It is the *pill* that can make you sleep. It has nothing to do with you, with your expectation of yourself.

Every successful night on medication means trust in oneself is diminished, and true recovery from insomnia becomes more remote. So even when sleeping pills succeed in making you sleep, they can never be successful in instilling a new habit and curing insomnia, because sleeping pills actually *reduce* one's expectation of being able to sleep unaided. So, once they have stopped working (as is the norm) the insomniac is cast adrift with no expectation of being able to sleep *at all*, with or without medication. As you may know, this is an extremely frightening place to find yourself.

Poor expectation is also the reason why other sleep aids may not work on you. People often write to tell me they have unsuccessfully tried all manner of herbs, recordings, mp3s, magnets, gizmos and gadgets. I personally must have tried over 100 different sleep aids during my 15 insomniac years. Why does none of them ever work? It is because most sleep aids work on tension levels, and nothing else.

The reason people so often say, 'Nothing ever works' is that nothing has ever made one jot of difference to their expectation. And every time they repeat this little sentence, 'Nothing ever works for me', that expectation weakens, the habit grows stronger and the insomnia becomes even more entrenched.

I sell brain entrainment mp3s on my website, but I go to great lengths to explain that listening to these recordings alone will be very unlikely to cure insomnia. Without also following the instructions in my books, there will be almost no chance of curing a moderate to severe problem. No matter how strong and high-quality the recording, even state-of-the art brain entrainment CDs will not overcome very low expectation. Low expectation is not something that can be 'cured' or fixed with one pill, one move, or one action. Expectation needs room and time to grow, to settle and to become habitual. Increasing expectation must be allowed to take as long as it needs and progress can be slow. In this book, I will be showing you the very best things you can do to speed up this process.

Let's recap this section:

IF ANXIETY IS TOO HIGH sleep will be hard to come by even if Expectation and Tiredness are high.

IF TIREDNESS IS TOO LOW sleep will be hard to come by even if Expectation is high and Anxiety is low

IF EXPECTATION IS TOO LOW, sleep will be hard to come by even if Anxiety is low and Tiredness is high.

Of course, you may have noticed that while I have separated tiredness, expectation and anxiety, this distinction is somewhat artificial. They are all so closely linked that they can be impossible to separate. These three aspects also feed and affect each other. Low expectation can cause anxiety. Anxiety in turn, feeds low expectation. Lack of tiredness will often increase anxiety and decrease expectation. Expectations are what inspire, feed and create one's actions and one's habitual behaviours, good and bad. Sometimes you may feel you are anxious because your thinking is negative and your expectation is low, and all of this serves to stop you feeling sleepy and tired enough to sleep, and that lack of tiredness just makes you feel more anxious, which shatters your expectation of being able to sleep! If you try to work it out, it fast becomes a jumbled mess. Little wonder insomniacs become obsessed with trying to work it out.

Let's go back to the TEA formula for good sleep. Remember: for good sleep, we must have optimum levels of:

TIREDNESS EXPECTATION ANXIETY

Now, really good sleepers don't attend to any of these things because:

- They go to bed when tired.
- They are naturally relaxed about sleep.
- And most of all, they have an absolutely cast-iron expectation that they will sleep.

This makes the association of bed and sleep absolute and so good sleep is utterly *inevitable*. They have such high levels of expectation that sleep comes without even having to think about it, without having to 'do' anything (like follow sleep hygiene rules or do a relaxation technique). For the good sleeper, sleeping is as automatic and unconscious as breathing. But here we have a dilemma. For insomniacs, sleep has become totally non-inevitable, totally conscious, and expectation is very low, which means there is *still* very much a need to 'do' something. In fact, the insomniac wants nothing more than to 'do something' to make things better again. But 'doing things' in bed only adds to self-consciousness; this makes going to bed and trying to sleep contrived, artificial, and a long way from being effortless. And for the person who is begging to be told what to 'do', it is no good just saying 'stop trying so hard' because that's like being told to stop thinking about the proverbial white bear.

So, how do we get from completely self-conscious, non-automatic, non-inevitable sleep (or no sleep) to unconscious, inevitable perfect sleep? How do we get to this level of unconsciousness, of 'inevitability' from a place which is very, very self-conscious, even obsessive?

Introducing
The Effortless Sleep Method

The Method laid out in *The Effortless Sleep Method* is a set of 12 promises I ask you to make in order to overcome insomnia. The first six promises are designed to sort out your *sleep hygiene*; in other words, your going to bed and in-bed habits. These promises are the more 'generic' bits of advice with which you may already be very familiar. They are designed to lay the ideal background, *physical* conditions which are most conducive to great sleep. Sleep hygiene works mainly to ensure that your anxiety and tiredness are at the ideal levels. By sorting out your sleep hygiene, you make things *easier* for yourself; you make it quicker and simpler to change the more difficult part of insomnia – your *habitual* negative thinking, your poor expectation.

The remaining promises are designed to work directly on this negative thinking. These will be quite unlike anything you will have heard before on any other sleep programme. Those of you who have already read *The Effortless Sleep Method* will also be very familiar with these.

Each one of these promises is designed to address *tiredness, expectation* or *anxiety* to produce the absolute ideal conditions conducive to good sleep. The combination of promises thus works on all three aspects, all at the same time. This may well be overkill for some people and you may end up attending to aspects that aren't really causing a problem. But doing this isn't going to make your sleep worse. The worst that any particular promise can do is nothing. The real advantage of this 'overkill' method is that it saves you from having to work out, analyse, and fret over which aspects are problems for you. In fact, it's essential you don't get bogged down, wasting time and attention deciphering which bits apply to your particular problem. You can tie yourself in knots with this sort of attention to detail. This is completely counterproductive and only serves to increase obsessive thinking.

You will probably also notice that many of these promises cover more than one aspect. Some cover all three. Sleep hygiene, while designed to make sure tiredness is at an optimum level, also increases expectation by strengthening the mental association of bed and sleep. And working directly on expectation will also usually reduce anxiety. This is another reason that it is not a good idea to pick out the promises you think are relevant and work exclusively on these. You may believe your tiredness levels are good, but if you thus ignore sleep hygiene, you then lose the benefits to your expectation and anxiety that some of these sleep hygiene-related promises afford.

It's also worth remembering that we insomniacs are notoriously bad at working out what our sleep problem is 'all about' and the best way to treat it. I'm usually in favour of the 'I know what's best for my body' approach, but with sleep this doesn't seem to hold. For example, for over ten years I resisted *all* forms of sleep hygiene, sure that it was the wrong approach. I was convinced it would add to my obsession, and that it would have no effect on a problem as bad as mine. Don't make the same mistake.

Give yourself the very best chance of recovery by working on *all* the promises.

And I must just mention this before I go on: Be sensible with caffeine. I don't include caffeine reduction as part of my programme because I don't want to insult anyone's intelligence. I assumed everyone knew that coffee, tea and cola contain large amounts of caffeine. I have since learned that a lot of insomniacs are drinking far too much caffeine without even realising. Remember, it's not just coffee that can cause a problem. Cola can be extremely stimulating, as can a strong cup of tea. You may think your after-dinner espresso is having no effect, but caffeine sensitivity can develop suddenly at any time. So, if you drink coffee, tea or cola after about 4pm, try cutting that out before you do anything else.

The 12 Promises

In the first book, I listed twelve promises. These have not changed. Each one of the promises of *The Effortless Sleep Method* is designed to address one or more of each of the components of the TEA formula.

Promise 1.

Spend less time in bed

(Tiredness)

Promise 2.

No naps

(Tiredness)

Promise 3.

Get out of bed when you can't sleep

(Tiredness, expectation, anxiety)

Promise 4.

Get up at the same time every day

(Tiredness, expectation)

Promise 5.

Do nothing in bed except sleep or have sex

(Expectation)

Promise 6.

Reduce or eliminate the pills

(Expectation, anxiety)

Promise 7.

Stop clockwatching

(Expectation, anxiety)

Promise 8.

Replace negative sleep talk with positive statements

(Expectation, anxiety)

Promise 9.

Let go of the search for an instant miracle cure

(Expectation)

Promise 10.

Discover a relaxation technique that works for you

(Anxiety)

Promise 11.

Decide on your own safety thought

(Anxiety, expectation)

Promise 12:

Put your life before your insomnia

(Expectation)

'I've had a quick look at the promises and I can tell you now: that's too simple. That's never going to cure my insomnia!'

Be warned, my books are not like diet books where the entire plan can be summed up on one page while the rest is case histories and 60 pages of recipes you'll never make. You'll soon discover that I don't do fluff and filler. I actually don't know how to write that way. Under no circumstances should you skip to the 'meat', to the cure section, read the list of promises and then declare 'that won't work'. That's like reading the table of contents or the index, and then declaring that book useless.

If you read these promises and find yourself disagreeing with any of them, or if you find you cannot understand why one of these promises is needed, please read the entire book first. And if you still don't believe this will work, go back and read the *The Effortless Sleep Method* where full explanation of the individual promises is given. And if you're still sceptical, then *stop reading* and just follow the instructions. Remember, I receive daily letters of thanks from people with problems just like yours. Many of them started off being highly sceptical of this method, sometimes having suffered for 30, 40 even 50 years. But all have overcome their insomnia using just the instructions in these two books.

'But spending LESS time in bed doesn't make any sense. Surely I should be trying to get as much sleep as I can?'

It might seem counterintuitive, but spending less time in bed is a recommendation I give to almost everyone. This promise has three distinct effects on sleep.

First, the less time you spend in bed, the less chance you have of lying in bed awake and so won't create a mental association of being in bed with being awake.

This means you will weaken the *expectation* of being unable to sleep in bed.

Second, if you are spending too long in bed, you are likely to doze, or get very light sleep without going into the deepest, and most refreshing, *delta* sleep. This results in your sleep 'thinning out' and so decreasing in depth and quality. By reducing your time spent in bed, you 'squash' the sleep into a tighter space, meaning the sleep you do get will be of better quality. If you are getting nine-plus hours of sleep but are still feeling lousy all day, getting less time in bed may well improve this.

Third, even though the replenishing effects of light sleep are minimal, large amounts of light sleep will still reduce your level of sleepiness when you next get into bed. By reducing the time you spend in bed, you slightly increase your tiredness levels and so make sleep easier to come by.

'But I don't know how many hours I need, or how much to cut down by.'

You will probably need to experiment to find your own ideal bedtime hours. A good rule is to start with the amount which seems right to you, minus half an hour. From now on, these 'bedtime hours' must be the maximum time and the *only* time you spend in bed.

'What's wrong with a nap? I have heard doctors say it's good for you. The Mediterranean countries always take a siesta and they are a very long-lived people.'

I'm sure a nap is good for you, if you live in southern Italy, have a leisurely paced life working in the sunshine, and don't have any sleeping issues. But that is not who you are. You are reading this book because you have an issue with insomnia, and things are slightly different for you; at least they will be in the beginning. (This goes for all those other things that normal sleepers do, such as reading in bed or having a sneaky lie-in at weekends.)

If napping in the day is the only decent sleep you get, it is *undoubtedly* at the expense of a proper full night's sleep. Even a 20-minute nap will mean that when you finally get to bed at night, you will be less sleepy than you would have been without it, making it more difficult to drop off. Additionally, taking a nap on the bus or train or sofa reinforces night-time insomnia by decreasing expectation of being able to sleep in bed.

'I'm really having a problem with promise 3 – 'getting out of bed when I can't sleep'. Do I REALLY have to do this? I think it stresses me out even more and might even be making things worse.'

Let's get one thing straight. You do not, and should not, need to jump out of bed the moment you wake in the night. I am *not* saying, like some other programmes do, that you should get out of bed after 20 minutes, or half an hour, or any such thing. The only promise you must make is that you get up *once you are wide awake.*

But what exactly does this mean? Exactly *when* should you get up? Well, the time is not important. In fact, if you have lain there for an hour, but still feel nice and drowsy and sleepy, like you could still fall asleep, it is probably better to stay where you are – sleep may still come yet. But if you are becoming more and more awake, or are wide awake, *get up.* You only need get up if you are becoming wide awake, or are starting to stress. The idea is that you avoid lying in bed in a stressed state, and so break the association of being in bed and anxious.

Remember, every minute that you lie in bed wide awake, you are strengthening the association of bed and being awake. You want the very act of getting into bed to make you start to fall asleep. This is how some people claim to 'fall asleep as soon as their head hits the pillow' – all they have different from you is an incredibly strong association between bed and sleep. You can create just such a trigger, but *not* if you lie around in bed not sleeping.

Also, you are more likely to fall asleep very shortly after getting into bed. If you go to bed, nice and sleepy, and then find that you have become awake again, it can take a very long time for the sleepy feeling to return. If you get out of bed, you can start the whole process all over again.

A time will soon come when you will no longer need to get out of bed, even if you do wake. These days, if I wake in the night, I just relax into the following safety thought, 'Oh goody, it's still dark. Lots of lovely sleep still to enjoy' and I go straight off to sleep again. It is very, very rare that I have to get out of bed these days.

If you do find yourself awake in the early hours, and find yourself becoming anxious, the best thing you can do is to get up and change your focus as soon as possible. Get yourself out of the drowsy, stressed 'I've-just-woken-up state', and do something else. Even having a bath or shower can be a good idea. But *whatever* you do, don't stress about the fact that you are out of bed. You shouldn't be focused on getting back into bed as soon as possible. Don't worry about the sleep you are missing in being out of bed; after all, you know that just one hour of really good deep sleep can be more refreshing than three or four hours of light sleep. By getting out of bed, you have a greater chance of getting that deep sleep. Remind yourself of that next time you wake at night, and you may find yourself much more relaxed about the whole thing. It will then be much easier to go back off to sleep.

People get more panicked about this sleep promise than any other. In some cases people have become so panicked that it is clouding everything and affecting their recovery. So these days, I allow transgression on this one promise, and the transgression must go like this: if you are really stressed about this one promise, then ignore it *for two weeks only*. All of the other promises *must* be followed exactly. If your sleep improves, fine: you can leave this promise out of your recovery programme. If it doesn't, and you still find yourself lying in bed fretting, then you *must* go back to getting out of bed. And don't decide to break this promise just because it doesn't work the first few times you try it. In the early days, this promise is *likely* to interfere with your sleep. You may even have a few sleepless nights *because* of it. But you should do your best to persevere. Remember, it isn't forever, it's just for now. This guideline is designed to break a negative association; it is not an insomnia cure in itself.

> *'I don't fancy having to get up really early at the weekends.*
> *I like to have a drink on Saturday night and Sunday morning is*
> *the only time I get any decent sleep.'*

Many people find that Sunday is the worst night of sleep for them. This can be down to the stress of returning to work, but there is something else at play. If you lie in bed until 11am on Sunday morning, come Sunday night you will not be particularly tired. This can set off another bout of insomnia, even when things have been going well.

It may surprise you to learn that I sell more books and CDs, have more website visitors and more emails on Monday and Tuesday than in the rest of the week put together. I can only assume it is down to the 'Sunday-night insomnia' phenomenon.

It may seem harsh not to allow a morning lie-in on Sunday, especially if the weekends are the only time you currently get any decent sleep. But *in the beginning,* it's very important to impose a moderately strict routine on your body. By getting one good lie-in a week, you could be sabotaging the other six nights. It's just not worth it.

'What if I have been awake all night? Am I still not allowed a lie-in?'

Lying in after a bad night is actually just another example of 'spending too long in bed'. Spending too long in bed is one of the worst behaviours an insomniac can have, causing a multitude of problems. We can summarise them here:

1. It reduces the quality of your sleep – causing it to 'thin out'.

2. By lying in bed just dozing you create more and more memories of the wrong kind – of the 'lying-in-bed-and-not-sleeping kind'.

3. It makes you less sleepy the following night and hence weakens your 'falling asleep response'.

4. It causes you to lie in bed stressing and becoming tense.

5. It is responsible for your thinking sleep is 'boring' or uncomfortable.

6. It sometimes adds to any depression by giving your mind the perfect time and opportunity to focus on all that is bad in your life.

7. It leaves you feeling *less* refreshed than a shorter time in bed.

Do I need to say any more?

My sleep is pretty near perfect now which means I can pay almost no attention to sleep hygiene at all. But, the one promise I almost always stick to is the 'not-lying-in-bed-in-the-morning rule'. I find a really long lie-in makes me feel bad all day. It's as if I can't shake off this heavy, bleary irritated feeling, even though I have slept a lot *more* than usual and even though much of this will be deep Delta sleep. To add insult to injury, I always find it takes me much longer to get to sleep the night after a long lie-in.

'But I'm naturally a "night owl". This means I find it really hard to get up early, especially when I don't have work in the morning.'

My partner is like this. He works late and finds it really hard to get up. He usually lies in bed, 'waking up', for at least another 30 minutes after the alarm has sounded. I am convinced that his lying around in bed is what causes him to a) have difficulty getting up in the first place and b) feel groggy and grouchy until about 11am! I know this because *it is how I used to be.* I was once exactly the same, hence my belief that I was not a morning person. I actually avoided doing 'proper' jobs for years just so that I could avoid getting out of bed in the morning.

It was my being an apparent 'night owl' which led me to self-employment, rather than ever having to suffer the horror of an early start at someone else's behest.

I can't believe how all this has changed. Now I *love* getting out of bed early.

This may sound a little excessive, but I almost leap out of bed when the alarm goes off. I wouldn't dream of pressing the 'snooze' button. I am up and sitting on the edge of the bed within seconds, almost before I have woken up! Then I sit there and 'catch my thoughts' until I become *compos mentis* enough to stand up. After a quick shower I go and get my morning coffee from a local cafe. That shower followed by a little walk in the morning air means that I am back home, wide awake, sharp as a tack and ready for anything *before my partner has even got out of bed!* Now, the reason this is easy for me is not because I am made of different stuff from him, *or from you*. It's just because I have done this so many times it has now become a habit. And once things become a habit, they become easy. In fact, anything else becomes difficult! I now love leaping out of bed. I hate that bleary morning feel and I want it gone as soon as possible. So why would I lie in bed and prolong the discomfort?

The key here is consistency. The more you do something, the easier it becomes, and it doesn't take many repetitions before it begins to feel like the norm. Try committing to getting up at the same time every day for 30 days. You will probably find that after about two weeks, it will have become close to a habit.

'I hear what you are saying, but I still might have trouble with getting up at the same time every day. I do shift work and so work irregular hours. Should I still try to go to sleep at the same time every night, and get up at the same time every morning?'

Shift-workers always have a tougher time on the programme than others. But it's not impossible to make it work by any means. You may find it near enough impossible to stick to getting up at the same time every day. In these cases, it is not absolutely essential to get up at exactly the same time every morning. What *is* essential is that you are tired when you lie down to sleep.

You may need to do a little experimentation and be a more flexible with your sleep patterns. For example, If seven-and-a-half hours is a good amount of sleep for you, then just make sure you only ever spend this time in bed. In other words, if you go to bed at 12, then get up at 7.30. If you go to bed at 2am, get up at 9.30. So just try to make sure you don't have more than seven-and-a-half hours in bed on any night. The idea is to get just the right amount of time in bed to make sure you are nice and tired when you lie down to sleep, while still being fresh and not unbearably tired during the day. If that means getting up a little later on one day than the previous, fine. You are doing the best you can.

Shift-workers also have sleep issues that are specific to their situation. For one, they tend to use tea, coffee and energy drinks to keep them going, perhaps even just a few hours before bed. If this is your tendency, it needs to stop.

Another common problem is finding it difficult to switch off when in bed. I hear shift-workers complain of this more than anyone. It seems the reason is simply this: after a nightshift, a worker often returns home exhausted, has a quick shower or bite to eat and goes straight to bed. But their mind is still completely wired and awake after work, even though physically their body is exhausted. Thus they are *tired* but not remotely *sleepy*. After a nightshift, or when going to bed at an 'odd' time, they don't have the usual winding-down routine and so don't give the normal signals to the brain and body that it's time to sleep. A worker will go to bed 'because it's time', but not follow the usual 'going to bed routine' that a normal night-time sleeper does. Think about it: a person working nine to five wouldn't dream of coming straight home and going to bed. They would come in, make some food, perhaps have a bath, watch a few hours of television or read, or even go out and see friends and watch a film, and *then* go to bed. All these simple things 'tell' the mind that it's getting toward bedtime. That way, the mind begins to wind down naturally and when bedtime comes, thoughts are fewer and the mind is calm.

So, the answer is *always* to try to stick to a normal winding-down and going-to-bed routine, no matter what the time is. This will prepare your mind nicely so that it 'knows' to expect bed and sleep. Try to do the same, peaceful enjoyable things every day before you go to bed, like reading, watching television, or something similar. Don't take a quick shower – take a long bath (if you have one), with *bubbles!* These activities should take up at least two hours of your time, to give the mind a chance to switch off.

If you are doing the kind of rotating shift pattern that consists of a week of nights followed by a week of days, then I probably cannot help you. I can't help you because you may not even have insomnia; you are just being tortured by your working hours. Much research has been done showing these work patterns to be very bad for physical and mental health. In my opinion these patterns are dangerous, unnatural and should probably be made illegal.

'Surely reading in bed is fine? Before my problem started I would always read to get me off to sleep.'

Reading in bed is a funny one. Some of the promises of my book are absolute. For example, I absolutely recommend reducing sleeping pills. I absolutely recommend stopping the negative sleep talk. These promises are universal, for everyone. But others are slightly more generalised. I can't pretend that reading in bed is harmful for every single insomniac. Some people find reading in bed really settles them down and is an important constituent in their pre-sleep routine. Plus, this is one of those promises that we don't want to be keeping *for ever*. Not reading in bed is, in effect, a small compromise to insomnia. (In fact, quite a few of my promises are compromises to insomnia.)

So, I will allow you to use your discretion with this one. If the thought of being able to read in bed gives you a sense of relief and relaxation, then by all means do it. It might mean that going to bed can be something to look forward to, rather than to fear, which is ideal. But, if it starts to affect your sleep, by resulting in your taking longer to fall asleep each night, then you may have to give it up again *for now*. In the beginning, we need to give you the very best chance of sleeping quickly and automatically. The idea is to create an association of bed–sleep that is so strong, it will overcome all the stresses and fears you may have that are preventing you from sleeping. That association will eventually become so strong that there will be no time for reading; you will be starting to nod off almost before you put your head on the pillow.

'Why are you so down on sleeping pills; if my doctor prescribes them, surely I ought to take them?'

First of all: you *must* get proper medical advice before starting any drug withdrawal programme. If you currently take a sleeping pill every night, particularly if it is a benzodiazepine or a Z-drug, then you *must* speak to your doctor first about giving it up. I am not a doctor, nor do I pretend to be. I may know about the psychology of insomnia but I have little professional or personal knowledge about the chemical and physical side-effects of withdrawing from your particular drug. This can be a dangerous process if not done correctly. *Don't take a risk; get advice.*

The aim of this programme is to rediscover and rekindle your own, natural ability to sleep. The taking of sleeping pills is in direct opposition to this approach. If you take a sleeping pill every night, you should speak to your doctor about reducing the dosage with a view to giving up altogether.

In *The Effortless Sleep Method* I described in detail the many negative side-effects of sleeping medications. I feel so strongly about this that one day I might even write a whole book on the subject. If you need convincing on this point in the meantime, you really should read my first book. To summarise: if you take a prescribed sleeping medication, you run the risk of developing addiction and many unpleasant physical and emotional problems. You may be more likely to crash your car, have accidents and your work and relationships may suffer. You may become depressed, anxious or even suicidal. You even increase the possibility of developing serious illness such as cancer and even your overall mortality risk is increased.

Now, hear this ... sleeping pills do *not* even make you sleep. That's right; they do *not* make you sleep. What they *do* is one of two things:

1. They knock you unconscious – not causing real, natural normal sleep, but drugged unconsciousness. There is *always* a high degree of hangover in this case, as the amount of genuine sleep obtained is minimal.

2. They give you faith and trust, which relaxes you enough to actually fall sleep – in effect, acting in a somewhat similar way to placebo. This is why some people, finding themselves awake in the early hours, are able to fall asleep *within seconds* of taking a pill. Similarly, those who take a tiny crumb of pill per night and find it effective, are also relying on little other than placebo. But, in this case, the pill does not have *no* effect, it just doesn't affect that which it is supposed to. The effect it does have is a negative one – feeling groggy and possibly anxious the next day.

I'm not down on pills because of some New Age self-righteous idea about 'naturalness' and avoiding 'drugs' because they are inherently 'bad' or sinful in some way. I say this because medications, both prescribed and over-the-counter, *do not cure insomnia.*

'But those nights with pills are the only nights I get any sleep at all. Can't I give them up once I start sleeping better?'

No. You have things backwards. The fact is, you won't start sleeping better *until* you give them up. How can you even *begin* to recover if you are reliant on drugs to make you sleep? Getting over insomnia is about learning to sleep 'like a normal person', without even thinking about it. It's about having complete trust in your own ability to sleep *on your own*. But this can't possibly happen if you are taking pills. Every time you take a pill you tell yourself 'I can't sleep'. In fact, you might as well say this affirmation every time you take a pill! Because that's the effect taking medication has. Every time you take a pill you deal another blow to the 'I'm a good sleeper' belief. In effect, you move further and further away from the beliefs you *do* want – *I'm a great sleeper, I can sleep on my own, I am getting better*, and move closer to and reinforce those rotten beliefs – *I'm an insomniac, I can't sleep on my own, I'll never get better.* Sleeping pills thus leave you with an absolute lack of faith in your own ability to sleep unaided, stripping you of that wonderful, childlike faith that allows the normal sleeper to sleep without thought or effort.

'But that is only true of those pills around at the moment. Sooner or later, doctors will invent a sleeping pill that DOES work. I'm looking forward to that day.'

Enjoy the wait. Because I'm not so sure there ever *will* be a sleeping pill that cures chronic insomnia, not *ever*. Think about it: good sleep is a delicate thing at the best of times. It is relatively easy to wake even a good sleeper. So even good sleep is *necessarily* delicate, fragile and easily disturbed. Good sleep needs to be 'real', not forced, and this sort of real sleep comes when you lie down, un-drugged, unaided, close your eyes and just go to sleep. That's what real sleep *is*. It is *necessarily unaided*. Unless you can learn to sleep like this, you will never get over your problem. Your mind, on the other hand, is strong. It is even strong enough, sometimes to keep you awake even when utterly exhausted, sometimes even through effects of the strongest sleeping pills. If you don't learn to sleep naturally and unaided, your mind will always be able to jump in and sabotage *any* external treatment, and so keep you awake. A large part of every chronic problem is to do with negative thoughts and beliefs. And until you address these beliefs, they will always be lying in wait, ready to sabotage any new treatment, drug or cure. You are still going to have easily disturbed sleep, you are still going to wake early during periods of stress and hence you are *still* going to have a problem *until* you fully address the beliefs aspect of your problem, no matter what new medications are rolled out.

New treatments may work for a bit, but only because you believe they will. But while your own trust in yourself remains low, it is only a matter of time before the treatment stops working and you are left with nothing.

If I had my way, sleeping pills would be renamed 'insomnia pills', because they do not make you sleep, and they cause more sleeping problems than they solve. I'd go as far as saying that if you are taking a daily sleeping pill, this is your *biggest* problem. In fact, I've said it before and I'll say it again: *sleeping pills actually make insomnia worse!*

'But I think I'm now addicted to the pills.'

Well, this is one area where I am afraid I must tell you to seek further help elsewhere. I can help alongside with the insomnia that may result from giving up, but you will need to seek professional advice from your doctor.

Sleeping pill addiction is a seriously nasty business and it can take many months or even years to fully get over it. The truth is, I was never even remotely addicted to sleeping pills. When I stopped any medication, I always did it suddenly without any complications other than rebound insomnia. Because of this, I cannot give the sort of intensely detailed advice that I do with insomnia, and legally I am simply not allowed to advise you.

All I see is the fallout, the victims. I can help support along the way, but you will need proper professional medical supervision. Asking your doctor for help doesn't *always* get a very supportive response. Doctors can sometimes be remarkably unwilling to agree with your decision to give up. But this is your body, and if you want to give up, it is your right to do so. Stick to your guns and demand support. And resist all pressure to 'try a new drug'. This is a common trick which *never* works in the long run.

If you have chronic insomnia, there is *not a single drug available that will cure you. Believe it!*

For more specific support, visit www.benzobuddies.com. While I do not advise visiting insomnia support forums, this one is a little different. The members there are really very helpful, are all dedicated to giving up the drugs, rather than just sharing horror stories, and they can help you through the dark times.

Be warned: there is a good chance that your insomnia will *worsen* for a time when you try to cut down. This is the well-documented 'rebound insomnia' which is a common side-effect of giving up sleeping medication. But it doesn't last forever and the final reward will make all those difficult nights worthwhile. You needn't cut back quickly. Take it as slowly as you like. You can reduce by one crumb of pill per week, if that makes things easier. And remember, every night on reduced medication is a triumph, *even if you do not sleep*.

I'll lay it on the line one last time: unless you cut back the pills with a view to giving up altogether, you will never, *ever* get over your insomnia, *ever!*

'How will I know how many hours I've slept if I don't look at the clock? How will I know I'm making progress?'

Now, one difference between mine and some other sleep programmes is that I do *not* advocate using sleep diaries, where every detail of one's sleeping and waking hours is recorded, in term of hours and minutes. I know that some people find them helpful. But for those who are trying to stop obsessing about sleep, keeping a sleep diary is a terrible reinforcing behaviour. All that really matters is how one feels, and how well one functions in the daytime. We have all had perfectly happy and productive days in the past after only a few hours' sleep. Obsessing about the number of hours we *ought* to be sleeping makes the possibility of these carefree days all the more unlikely.

Clockwatching only creates an unhealthy obsession with time. From now on, I want you to pay *no* attention to the number of hours of sleep you get. Work out how many hours you need, set your getting up time and from then on, *forget about time*. From now on, you should have *no idea* how many hours you slept last night. All that matters is how well you feel during the day.

This is particularly important for sleep-maintenance insomniacs. By watching the clock and being aware of the time you create strong 'wake-up anchors' in your mind. Remember, your mind and body already have a very strong sense of what time it is (the 'internal clock'). If you look at the clock when you wake and find it is usually around 2am, for example, this pattern becomes reinforced. Eventually, 'I always wake at 2am' becomes close to a *fact* in your mind. This makes the pattern very hard to break.

It may surprise you to know that I, too, wake up most nights simply to use the loo. But, being perfectly honest with you, I have no idea whatsoever when this happens, I just know that it does. It could be 1am, it could be 6am. Unless it is getting light, I really don't know. And after using the loo, I am asleep again within minutes. But if I started watching the clock, and came to realise that I was waking every night at 2am, I would be in trouble. Before long, I would become so aware of this time, that this knowledge would spill over into my waking life, becoming more and more strongly believed. It would soon become a hard *fact* that I get up every night at 2am. *Then* I would have a real problem, one which is suddenly much harder to deal with.

If you have sleep-maintenance insomnia, you wake too early and cannot get back to sleep. This is your type of insomnia, this is your problem, *this is your story*. By taking away all knowledge of when you have woken up, immediately that story loses some of its power; it becomes less convincing, less factual, less set in stone.

The belief that you 'wake every night at around 2am' has already been weakened, just by the one small move of avoiding looking at the clock.

'I'm trying to replace negative sleep thoughts with positive ones. But I find this really difficult. It seems I have no control over my negative thoughts and I still have a lot of fear and worry in this area.'

A large part of this book is dedicated to answering exactly this question so read on.

'Why do I have to let go of the search for a cure? I think it makes sense to keep on trying new remedies. If I keep at it, eventually I'm bound to find the one that works, aren't I?'

In the first book I describe the terrible personal laboratory where we become the subject of our own miserable, pointless experiments into sleeping problems. I have some people who write regularly to tell me about the latest new relaxation programme they have started, or the umpteenth therapy course they have taken. No matter how many times I tell them that this is counterproductive, they don't seem to get it.

How can you believe you are getting over your problem, if you are still dedicating so much time to looking for a cure? Every time that you search for another cure or try the latest sleeping pill, you are saying to yourself, 'I have a problem', 'I fear insomnia', 'I don't believe I can sleep' and so push that recovery further and further away.

'Promise 10 may be difficult for me. I am a very anxious person and find it difficult to relax. Can you give me any pointers?'

This is such an important subject that I'm going to dedicate the following large section to it.

Dealing with Stress, Tension and Anxiety

Almost all of us are suffering from too much stress. And most of us have worries, niggles, neuroses and obsessions. I did when I suffered with insomnia, and I still do. We are all told to do something about reducing stress, taking time out for ourselves, recharging our batteries, but how many of us really make stress reduction a priority in our lives? Most of us have come to take stress for granted, just to accept it as an inevitable part of life.

But stress is a real killer of good sleep. It can cause you to have difficulty falling asleep, cause you to wake too early, and the sleep you do get will often be of poor quality.

Some people are able to deal better with stress than others, and if you suffer badly with stress, you really must find a way to deal with it. Insomnia is likely to be only one of a whole host of symptoms that may start to show themselves as physical illness or emotional problems. Bizarrely, it is often those who are most stressed who complain they are 'unable to relax' and so ignore all advice to do so. If you are one of those who find it really difficult to relax, you *of all people* need to find a way. It is essential, for your sleep and for your well-being in general. If your job, for example, is causing you to lose sleep on a regular basis, you must do one of two things if you don't want to end up in a very bad place indeed. Either sort out your stress levels so that you are able to deal with things better, or get a new job! No job is worth chronic insomnia.

'But whenever I use any relaxation method, it wakes me up even more!'

You may already have noticed that night-time relaxation is not quite as straightforward for insomniacs as it is for normal sleepers. Most insomnia advice will involve techniques designed for 'what to do in bed when you can't sleep'. But if you're a chronic insomniac, you may find yourself unwittingly fighting any 'in-bed' technique or a relaxation recording, particularly if it is new and unfamiliar. If you're a 'fighter' you may have found CDs, mp3s and relaxation techniques useless.

Insomniacs also tend to obsess about the way they feel, and focus on tiny little nuances of their emotion and bodily sensations as they try to relax. This is why many people find that, far from helping, night-time techniques actually 'wake them up'.

It can be very tempting to treat a relaxation method, CD or recording as a cure in itself. Sometimes, people buy my Sleep Tools and then email to say, 'They need to be here by Friday because I have an important day on Saturday and I simply *must* get some sleep the night before!' Some even *wait* until a high-pressure night to test the new CD (this was my mistake for years).

These people have almost no chance of success. The erroneous thought behind these actions is that it is the relaxation method that is making you sleep. It isn't. Not ever. All a relaxation method ever does is calm you down enough to *let yourself* sleep.

Have you ever tried a sleep aid, my Sleep Tools or some other method and approached it thinking something like this? 'This is going to work tonight, it *has* to work tonight, *please* God, Jehovah, Allah, Buddha make it work tonight!'

So you lie down; your anticipation is immense and your heart is pounding. You begin to relax a little, becoming a little drowsy. Perhaps, just maybe, this is actually going to work tonight. You wait … nothing…you wait some more, painfully aware of waiting for the results of your experiment. Just this awareness of being aware seems to be enough to keep you awake. You wait some more, waiting for the relaxation to return … and wait … and wait. And then it happens … the little 'jump' – the little lurch, or leap into wakefulness. Eventually the horrible, dawning realisation comes over you – I'm not sleeping. Please, not tonight! Not again! It is at this point that many people turn to sleeping pills.

This is all wrong.

Generally speaking, if you wait until bedtime to deal with high stress, you are going to be in trouble. This is simply a case of leaving things until too late. On those high-pressure nights, if you are tense and wound up when you go to bed, with fearful thoughts of not sleeping, with your heart thumping as you begin to undress, there is not a thing on this planet short of a sledgehammer that is going to make you sleep. Because of these issues, it really is so much more important and effective to deal with reducing your general background stress *during the day*. This is also easier than trying to de-stress at night because there is no pressure to actually fall asleep. With no extra 'agenda' of needing to be asleep at the end of it, the relaxation will actually be more successful.

Moreover, if you work on reducing stress throughout the day, there may well be no need to use a technique when bedtime comes and sleep can be much closer to the automatic, inevitable sleep which is our goal. When you get into bed, you will know there is nothing to try and think, nothing to try to 'do', nothing to get right. All that needs to be done *has been done* earlier on in the day. There is no point in any fretting, any wondering, any *doing*. Thus tension will be lower, *expectation of sleep will be higher*, thoughts are dreamier and sleep comes so much more easily. Do this well enough and sleep will be automatic!

And if you *do* enjoy using a night-time technique, it will be so much more effective if you are already half-way there.

How to Chill Out in the Day

Meditation Will Change Your Life

We are constantly being told about the virtues of meditation. *We should put time aside for silence. We should quieten our minds. We should learn to live in the moment* ... you've heard it all before. However, when I suggest you take up meditation this should not be rejected as generic 'you-just-need-to-chill-out' advice.

Daily meditation can have an astonishing, almost immediate effect on anxiety levels. Take up daily meditation and even high levels of anxiety could become a thing of the past. 'Deep-seated issues' will bother you less, and you may find new insights regarding them. The most common effect of meditation is that people report 'not being bothered about things so much'. Life just becomes subtly easier and easier, freer and lighter.

If you fancy learning, look for a local class, buy a book or CD or just follow the instructions for meditating in *The Effortless Sleep Method*. You could also do an internet search and find similar basic instructions.

I started out by learning Transcendental Meditation (TM) many years ago. This involves meditating with a mantra – a meaningless word which does not stimulate thought, but acts as a place to 'rest' your attention and so calm your mind. TM needs to be done twice a day for 20 minutes each time. I then moved to Buddhist-style 'watching the breath', and finally Zen-style 'doing nothing'. (Note that you do *not* need to have any part of the religious or spiritual side to practise meditation.)

But more recently I have taken to 'cheating' by using a meditation recording. If you don't have the discipline or time for twice-daily meditation, you also can 'cheat' by using one of these recordings. I did Holosync for years, but although the quality of recording was excellent, my progress was slow. More recently, I have taken to using a similar product called called BrainEV, which, for me, has a more rapid and noticeable effect. I like to listen to BrainEV while also using a mantra. This results in a *profoundly* deep and delicious meditation which I find utterly blissful. You can download a completely free trial recording at www.brainev.com. It's fun and easy to use and takes no effort whatsoever. Within a few months or even weeks, you could feel like a different person.

Another great thing about using a recording is that you do not need a perfectly silent house in which to meditate. Your husband can be banging around in the kitchen, your kids can be watching television in the next room … and you can just close the door, put on your headphones and be in a different world in minutes.

Alternatives to Meditation

If meditation really isn't your thing you could try yoga. Or, if you can afford it, have an essential oil massage three times a week.

If you really don't know where to start with a day-time relaxation method, just try seriously increasing your exercise levels. Did you know that exercise combined with meditation has an effect on sleep, anxiety and depression so good it blows the result for antidepressants out of the water? (And it makes you look good too!)

There are also several products and methods I recommend which you can find online. Every product I recommend in this book is one that I personally used and found helpful in overcoming insomnia. But not every technique is good for every person and you will need to experiment with different techniques for yourself.

For me, it was important that the technique I used had at least some instant effect. I always recommend tapping (www.emofree.com) and The Sedona Method (www.sedona.com) for this reason. Both have an 'in-the-moment' effect which means you can be feeling calmer, lighter or more positive immediately.

I sell my own range of Sleep Tool recordings which use a similar technology to Holosync and BrainEV. It's important to remember that these Sleep Tools act as a supplement to the instructions in my books. They will *not* cure insomnia in themselves and in no way *replace* following the Method, but they can really add a boost to the effect of the promises and they provide an easy and enjoyable way to relax. No technique or recording is likely to help if the other commitments are not in place. As a reader of my books, you can get these at a discounted price by visiting www.sashastephens.com/discount.

*'But what about the nights? What should I do if
I just find myself lying there, unable to sleep?'*

Sometimes your thoughts and anxiety just get the better of you. Sometimes you will get to bedtime and find yourself panicking. Sometimes you will find yourself with an obsessive negative thought that you just can't shake off. And what you probably want to know is how to deal with this sort of problem when it happens, *in bed at night*.

So, what are the best techniques?

Sorry to become a little hazy in my advice, but when it comes to night-time, this is very much a personal affair. There is no 'right' answer, no 'ideal' technique. This is something you much experiment with. For example, I know many people have a lot of luck with progressive relaxation, moving slowly through the body, relaxing one body part at a time. Not me. I find this completely useless. You may be different. Many people swear by my Sleep Inducer mp3 recording. Some have found using tapping or The Sedona Method very helpful to do when lying in bed.

Some people like to do little visualisations, they imagine themselves filling with heavy sand, or floating pink light, or that they are relaxing onto a magical cloud, or that a sleep angel is watching over them …

When I wake up in the night and get up to use the toilet, I tend to use a little visualisation to get me back off to sleep. For example, that I have been lost in the woods, stumbling in the dark, exhausted until I come across a perfect little magical hut, and inside it is the safest, most comfortable bed in the world. And as I actually get back into bed and lie down, I imagine myself lying down into this wonderful imaginary bed. But this visualisation is entirely personal to me. It is something *I* find incredibly delicious and soothing. This is important because by making it a really fun and enjoyable visualisation, I can do it just for its own sake. I do it for fun, because I like it. The fact that it helps me sleep is just a welcome side-effect. If you decide to try a visualisation, you should also make sure it is one that is personal to you, something you would do because you enjoy the experience. If you do experiment with visualisation, realise that the point is not to focus hard. If your mind starts to wander to something completely unrelated, *let it.* Focusing hard on anything is likely to keep you awake. Note that I rarely use this sort of visualisation for actually falling asleep in the first place. I too, find that doing anything in bed 'to make me sleep' often has the opposite effect. If visualisation doesn't work *at all* for you, don't worry. This is a very common complaint.

****

Technique: My Absolute Favourite Insomnia-Killing Relaxation Regime

The following is a wonderful practice which will make a profound difference to your sleep and your life in general. Meditate *twice* a day using a mantra or watching the breath, for 20 to 30 minutes, morning and early evening. Twice a day works *far* better than just once and has way more than double the effect of a single meditation! Then, at bedtime, meditate sitting in bed in the darkness for just a few minutes until you feel yourself starting to nod off. Gently lie down, paying no attention to anything in particular. Just lie there, do nothing and let your thoughts drift. This practice will often allow a person to fall asleep almost instantly and it was after doing this that I had my first ever experience of 'being asleep before my head hit the pillow'.

****

I know I have been a little vague in my advice regarding bedtime relaxation. But this vagueness is intentional. The reason I tell you to 'find a relaxation method that works for you' is to make you aware of just how personal a matter this is. It is very important you realise that if a particular technique doesn't work well for you, this is in no way a reflection of the severity of your problem, nor does it indicate that you are broken or different in some way.

So to recap, when it comes to relaxation, remember:

1. Don't make the mistake of 'testing' a technique on a high-pressure night.
2. You should use any new recording or technique until it has become very familiar.
3. If it doesn't work one night this doesn't mean it won't work on another night.
4. No technique, sleep aid or relaxation method works for all people.
5. Daytime de-stressing activities are often more effective than night-time relaxation techniques.
6. No relaxation method, CD or recording should be seen a cure in itself.

'You have told me to use a safety thought in bed when I can't sleep. But I'm not sure I know what you mean by a "safety thought".'

External crutches like sleeping pills and special pillows give you a safety net, something to believe in, and something to trust when you feel anxious. A safety thought is just my phrase for a 'safe thought' – a *fact*, something true that has happened, or something you believe, which calms and soothes you when you are worried about whether you will sleep. This might be along the lines of 'I can have a good day tomorrow even if I don't sleep' or 'I slept last Wednesday when I didn't expect to, so I can do the same tonight.' When the panic comes over you and thoughts of not sleeping fill your head, you simply need to remind yourself of your safety thought.

Can you remember a night, or a stretch of nights when you slept really well? Can you remember a time when you didn't expect to sleep and yet still did? Try to find a comforting and encouraging *fact* about your sleep. Have you had even *one* good night's sleep recently? Pick whatever positive fact you feel would be most likely to give you hope. When you lie down at night, relax into the comfort of your safety thought and let it soothe you.

If you find this promise particularly difficult, you should do the special 'Belief-Changer Technique' later in the book which will make a safety thought much easier to find.

'But there seems to be a contradiction here. You tell us to put our lives first, and not to make compromises for the sake of sleep. For me, that means going to bed whenever I like, reading where I like, and not compromising my life with all these "promises".'

Later in the book, I will tell you all about moving past insomnia, sleep hygiene and all compromise. Once your sleep improves, you can be looser with the sleep hygiene and you can let go of many of these promises. Eventually we will get you to that place of acting and thinking like a normal good sleeper. But don't try to run before you can walk.

For *now*, your sleep will be far too fragile to cope with so little discipline. It's far better to make things easy for yourself in the beginning by giving your sleep a little structure, a little order and a little stability. Even these days, if ever I have a less than perfect night, or I'm under particular stress, I immediately implement stricter sleep hygiene. This gives my sleep just enough of a push to get me back on track in no time.

'I'm doing my very best to stick to the promises, but I keep making little mistakes and getting really stressed about it. I'm never sure if I'm getting things right.'

You need to realise that each of these promises, and even all of them together, do not *make* sleep happen. Nothing can do that. What these promises do is to ensure that tiredness, expectation and anxiety are at optimal levels. They thus lay the groundwork, the ideal conditions for sleep to occur naturally, effortlessly.

You should never set out to break your promises. But if you get one little bit 'wrong' occasionally, that's fine as long as you can still cast it in a positive light. Never beat yourself up for the odd slip-up. Just refocus and get back to the programme. In fact, I think it's important that there be some flexibility. Stick to the programme but not too vehemently.

'Okay, now I'm really confused. Am I supposed to follow your rules or not?'

First of all, they are *not rules*, they are promises. I intentionally avoided calling these 'rules' with good reason. There is only a small difference between commitment and trying too hard. There is taking advice, and there is religiously obsessing over the details of that advice. There is being motivated to change, and being frantic to change. There is sticking to the programme, and there is being constantly preoccupied with the programme. If you stick too vehemently to the promises, one little slip-up is going to leave you feeling lost and despondent. *This* is why I avoid talk of rules.

Follow my instructions, yes. But if you do this while fussing over whether you are getting it exactly right, *then you are not getting it right*. Can you see this?

> *'I have heard about sleep hygiene before. But you must understand, I have suffered for decades. I don't think avoiding naps and having no clock in the room is going to work with a problem as bad as mine.'*

But have you simply read about sleep hygiene, or have you actually, properly (and I *mean* properly, not for just a couple of nights) tried it? Have you made it part of your life for a sustained period of time? Or have you read about it, picked out the bits you liked, tried it for a night or two and then rejected it as too basic and simple to help with your particular problem?

There is a reason that all insomnia books contain sleep hygiene – it is because sleep hygiene is *essential* to recover from insomnia. Does this mean that sleep hygiene alone will cure chronic insomnia? No, of course not. This is why both of my books are over 180 pages long.

> *'But you don't seem to understand. I've tried this before without much success. You have to admit that sleep hygiene rules are less important for chronic, long-term insomniacs, aren't they?'*

Absolutely *not!* Many long-term insomniacs will have tried sleep hygiene before, but without attention to their expectation, attitude, thoughts and beliefs, they will have had little chance of making any real progress. This is why sleep hygiene is often rejected by chronic insomniacs as something else that 'didn't work'. While chronic insomnia is always more of a thoughts-and-beliefs problem, it will be near enough *impossible* to overcome chronic insomnia if sleep hygiene is poor. So make things easy on yourself. Lay the foundation for the other promises to work their magic. Stop saying you've heard it all before and *do it*.

The fact is, *both* sleep hygiene and attention to thoughts are essential to beating insomnia. Asking which is more important is like asking which is more important to losing weight, diet or exercise. Of course, the answer is both. You *can* lose weight by dieting alone, but if you are lying in front of the television 24 hours a day, you will have a tough time making progress. Similarly, you can do load of exercise, but if you eat junk the moment you get out of the gym, progress will be tough. It's exactly the same with sleep hygiene and positive thinking. If you want to give yourself the best chance of success, do them both.

So, there you go. That's the Method. That's all you need to cure insomnia. You now have the exact instructions that have allowed tens of thousands of people to overcome their sleep problems. Off you go and start sleeping brilliantly!

> *'But we are less than half way through!*
> *What's the rest of the book for?'*

Okay, let's take one step back.

You may have read my first book and felt great afterwards. You may even feel that now. You may have that self-help book buzz and feel capable of anything. I know this feeling all too well.

From now on, *it's all going to be different!* You are *going to beat this.* You understand, *finally.* You know what to do, *finally.* And you may feel that nothing on earth could bring you down. But if I abandoned you in this state, I would be absolutely negligent in my job as a sleep therapist, because only half the job is done. No matter how positive you feel right now, sooner or later, things *are going to take a turn for the worse.* When you next miss a night … that's right, *when,* not *if,* you next miss a night, you need to be fully prepared. If not, you will go to pieces, let all the good intentions go, give up all the good behaviours, my Method will go on the scrapheap, and you will once again be on your own.

> *We need to act now before the next bad night hits.*

It is to this subject that we now turn

Cℬ

Stage Three
Repairing
When it All Goes Wrong …

'IT'S ALL GONE WRONG! I was feeling so positive after reading your book. I used the Method and it worked great for a few days/weeks/months. But then last night out of the blue it stopped working and my insomnia is back.'

'What to do when it goes wrong' is the issue that bothers most people. Almost all of my consultations are taken up by answering versions of this question. For many people, this section may well be the most important of the book.

Many people diligently follow my instructions, and have great success for a few weeks or even *months*. But then the Method apparently 'stops working' for one, two or more nights and the sufferer inevitably claims that their 'insomnia is back', or that they have suffered a terrible 'relapse'. Most people find it relatively easy to stay positive when they have slept well, but the moment a bad night comes along, they let all those good thoughts go out of the window and they feel back at square one. If this happens to you, be sure to come back and read this section again.

Now listen carefully …

What you are experiencing is *absolutely normal*. It's not only normal, it's *expected*. Occasionally, people write to say they have cured their insomnia instantly with my methods. But this is rare. More often than not, what they experience is something very like the situation I have just described: an initial success, followed by a little period of poor sleep.

What almost every other insomnia book leaves out, what doctors and therapists often don't acknowledge or recognise, is that getting over insomnia does not just involve sleeping better. It also involves learning to cope *when you don't*. I suspect that the only reason many other sleep cures and programmes are unsuccessful is because they don't give you proper advice about what to do *when* things go wrong. This little bit of poor sleep is actually completely irrelevant in terms of your overall recovery. The thing that will ensure you become a winner in the fight against insomnia is *what you do from this point on*. Because, *more than anything*, it is how you react when that happens that will determine how successful you are in overcoming insomnia.

If you work *only* on the first aspect – sleeping better, and judge progress based solely on this, you will have a *much* harder time, your recovery will be slower and you may never properly recover at all.

Why is this?

It is because one night, sooner or later, you will not sleep …

That's right … sooner or later, you will have a really bad night …

In fact I *promise and guarantee* that you will miss more nights …

Now, if you aren't prepared for bad nights, and you don't deal with them properly when they occur, then those bad nights will continue to plague you, fear of them will continue to haunt you and the threat of another bad spell of insomnia will always be imminent. And, with this fear hanging over you, full recovery will remain elusive.

'But it was going so well. I must have done something wrong, mustn't I?'

In the early days bad nights *will* come along for seemingly no reason whatsoever. And it is completely pointless to keep looking at what you did wrong, or what you could have done differently. There are all sorts of reasons why you may miss a night's sleep. You may have had a slightly more stressful day, your hormone levels are ever so slightly different, you ate different food, drank different drink, you are slightly hungry, dehydrated … who knows? The insomniac starts off as extra-sensitive to such things, and so is badly disturbed by little things which may not affect a good strong sleeper. This is why a few poor *nights are to be expected, especially in the beginning.*

And please realise, even the very best sleepers will occasionally sleep badly. Even *I* sometimes still sleep badly – usually because I have been working too late into the night, but sometimes for no reason at all. It is actually impossible to work out just why this happens. But whereas the normal sleeper just shrugs this off, drinks an extra cup of coffee, gets on with the day and forgets about it, the insomniac can only think one thought: the insomnia is back again! Panic, fear, 'Oh no, no, no!'

Both the good and the bad sleeper have experienced exactly the same thing: they both have missed a night's sleep.

But whereas the bad sleeper panics and declares, 'Insomnia is back again', the good sleeper doesn't even have the word 'insomnia' in their vocabulary.

I want you to give up all thoughts of never again missing a night's sleep. Not just because it's inevitably going to happen but because acceptance of this fact is going to be vital to your recovery. If you can really take this point on board, you will have acquired one of the very most important beliefs of all in overcoming insomnia, something which will be worth its weight in gold over the coming weeks and months.

Accept it: sleep patterns and success almost always go up and down. No one sleeps perfectly every single night of their lives, and no one gets no sleep at all, night after night. It is very, very important to understand, believe and accept this. Because if you are fully prepared and accepting of the fact that another bad night *will* come, it will end up being nothing but a blip. Indeed, bad nights can be a *blessing* if you respond to them well. If you can have a really bad night of sleep but remain positive, buoyant and full of hope, this night will add *infinitely* more to your recovery than a great night of sleep. After all, everyone can feel good and positive after a *good* night. It is your handling of these occasional *bad* nights and bad stretches that will really accelerate your progress.

So, paradoxical though it may sound, rather than do all in your power to avoid bad nights, *you actually need to experience a few of them!*

'But you don't know what it's like for me. It's not possible for me to feel positive when I haven't slept. I try to feel good, really I do. But as soon as I have a bad night it's like a switch goes on. None of the usual positive thinking seems to work and I can't feel happy again until I get some sleep.'

Rest assured, I know absolutely how bad it feels for you. I once had an almost phobic reaction to a bad night of sleep, 'plunging into an instant pit of despair', as I liked to describe it. Once upon a time, I would get up from a sleepless night in utter misery, spend the day desperate, panicky and tearful, wondering why, oh why, oh why I couldn't get over this bloody insomnia!

Believe me, there was a time when I would have wanted to punch anyone who suggested that missing sleep was not a problem. People would often say, 'Yeah, I sometimes don't sleep either; it's no big deal'. My goodness, how *ignorant* these people were! Didn't they understand? It was *different* for me!

So you see: *I do get it*. I do get why you find it difficult or impossible to avoid going to pieces every time you miss a night. And because I get it, please accept that what I am telling you is the truth. There is nothing necessary about the connection between lack of sleep and misery. This reaction, too, is simply a habit. You have simply become stuck in a habitual thought pattern that says 'lack of sleep means misery'. In my case, it was by taking control of that habitual reaction, just a *tiny* bit (for example by distracting myself with activities, 'pretending' I was feeling okay when really I wasn't, or by being 'okay' with the low mood and not beating myself up for it) that I began the task of turning my problem around.

My son Robin, who is 24, often spends a whole night partying and then goes to work the next day, with no ill effects whatsoever; it doesn't even affect his mood. I recently met Robin for morning coffee in the cafe where I sometimes write. He is a brilliant portrait tattoo artist but likes to paint in his spare time. A local bar had commissioned him to paint a mural on the wall of their main room. But as the bar is open all day, the only time that Robin had to paint was during the night, from 2am to 9am. So, in order to fit the commission into his timetable, he *chose* to stay up all night painting, after a full day's tattooing at his studio. That morning, he was in his usual jovial mood, joking, smiling, upbeat. Did he not feel exhausted, I asked? 'Yes,' he laughed. 'I feel like I'm floating. I quite like it.' He then went on to his studio, did a short day, sticking needles into people's arms without any accidents, and went to bed at a normal hour.

Now why can't we all be like that? Why is it that a missed night sends us into a pit of misery and panic? There isn't something fundamentally different about my son. He isn't 'made' of different stuff; he doesn't have some special ability. It just doesn't cross his mind to worry about missing a night of sleep. And *this* is why he doesn't feel bad. Of course, he feels tired. He feels *exhausted*. But he doesn't add worry, tension, anxiety and panic to the tiredness. So it's just tiredness, nothing more.

You can develop a similar outlook. Of course, when we are very tired, we aren't going to feel at our sparkling best. We may be groggy, less energetic, a bit more irritable. But this does not mean we have to fall into panic, depression and despair.

You need to find a way to accept, to *believe*, that the reaction to a bad night is, to a certain extent, a *choice*. I know from *bitter* personal experience that this is easier said than done. But that does not mean it *can't* be done. It takes a bit of repeated effort, that's all. If I had continued to fall apart and weep every time I slept badly, I would never have ended up in my current happy place.

Next time you get a bad night, resolve, to the best of your abilities, to have the best day you possibly can.

But I feel physically bad when I haven't slept, really terrible. My eyes hurt, my head aches, and I am stiff all over. Sometimes I feel dizzy and faint and even nauseous. It's impossible to forget about the fact I have missed a night's sleep when the way I feel physically reminds me all day.'

Once again, this need not be an automatic response. I am still amazed myself at how much tension levels and worry affect the actual, qualitative *feel* of lack of sleep. I believe it is this tension and worry that are largely responsible for the various physical symptoms that often follow after a bad night. The following incident from my own life will illustrate just how extreme these physical reactions can be.

Most chronic insomniacs have a few really bad experiences as a result of insomnia. Many of us have a horror story. Perhaps the time you burst into tears in a meeting, fainted at a wedding or just an important event that was so marred by exhaustion that you made a complete fool of yourself, or you just went through a complete day of hell, physically and emotionally.

I have one of these.

When I was at my craziest, I was going out with a naval officer at the time and went to a Royal Navy ball. It was a very elegant event and I needed to be on my best sparkling behaviour, witty and beautiful. But I had not slept the night before and had been stressing and fussing all day. By the time I reached the ball, I was close to hysteria. I had worked myself into such a state of pitiful, panicky exhaustion that after a short time, I escaped to the loos, where I had a violent vomiting attack (and I am someone who is almost never sick) and then collapsed. I had to be helped by the toilet attendant. It was so embarrassing. I had to leave this wonderful evening and return, weeping, to my hotel. I thought I had gone mad. I really thought the men in white coats would be coming to get me in the morning. But, I got through it. And now I'm saner than I have ever been.

So why am I telling you all this? Well, it's not so we can share and commiserate! It's because, looking back, I realise that this extreme *physical* reaction had very little to do with a lack of sleep, and everything to do with my way of dealing with it. It was caused, not so much by the lack of sleep, but by my stress and anxiety *about* the lack of sleep. Because since then, I have missed many, many nights where lack of sleep has hardly bothered me. Earlier this year there was a night when I was kept awake almost all night by my partner, who had a bad attack of food poisoning and was back and forth to the loo every few minutes. I slept maybe half an hour, and was awake from 3am until I got up. The next day I was exhausted, almost in a dream from lack of sleep. But, because this *wasn't a case of insomnia*, there was none of the misery, the worry, the depression. And more recently, there was a night where I was up all night working on a case of copyright infringement. This was quite a stressful night for me. The next day, I was tired, *just tired*, that's all. I wasn't at my best by any means, but I wasn't unhappy in any way.

Often, the terrible way we feel is less about lack of sleep itself, and more about *our reaction to it*, and we can learn to control that reaction. I am now able to miss nights *relatively* easily. I get up feeling rough, but after a coffee and some food and a bit of exercise, I feel better. By lunchtime I have usually forgotten that I had even missed the night's sleep! This seems incredible when I think of how it used to affect me. A missed night's sleep would once have sent me into a pit of depression and panic, even creating physical symptoms like sinus headaches, sore throat, tummy aches and strange aches in my hips and shoulders. Now I just shrug off a bad night. This is what has made me realise that it is the fear, the tension, the worry that is the *real* killer, *not* the lack of sleep per se.

You may also find that when you have had a bad night before something fun or important, you find yourself obsessively focusing on the way you feel, constantly thinking, 'I would enjoy this *so* much more if I didn't feel so tired.' I would sometimes find that even after a *good* night I was so used to focusing on the way I was feeling, that I would *still* find myself checking constantly. 'Am I tired, could I feel better, shall I meditate, do I need more coffee? Should I attempt a nap?' And the funny thing was, because I had been stressing so much about how I was feeling, by the evening I would often feel almost as bad as I had when I had missed sleep!

Unbelievable though it may seem, most of what you are feeling on a really bad day is actually tension and worry.

'But you aren't telling me how to overcome insomnia, just to accept it or pretend it isn't there. I don't want to accept insomnia. I don't want to "learn to live with it". I want to be RID of it!'

So, you think I've really copped out here; I've cheated. I'm supposed to be telling you how to sleep better. But instead of telling you how to sleep better, all I do is tell you to stop making a fuss when you *don't* sleep! That's a bit of a con, isn't it?

No. Don't you get it? The reason I am banging on about this 'being positive about the way things are' is not so that you just become 'okay' with the status quo. I don't want just to teach you how to *cope* with your current problem.

On the contrary: the fact is that by learning not to care so much about your *current* problem, your *current* problem will start to improve!

If you are in the throes of chronic insomnia, 'being okay with your current situation' will seem out of the question. But this is not a small point you can pass over. You cannot reject this part of the plan as 'impossible for someone like you'. This is *absolutely* the turning point to recovery. When you can really be okay with the fact that you will get a bad night from time to time, not only do those bad nights not worry you so much, *but they actually stop occurring so often!* The key to your recovery, the key to almost every long-term insomniac's problem, is to foster a way to not mind so much about missing sleep.

Not minding so much about whether you sleep is probably the one single most important change in attitude that you can make.

Because, it is the panic over not sleeping on the *first* night that turns *one* night into *two* nights, and *two* nights into a bad stretch. The way to break out of this fear–insomnia–fear cycle is to really realise and accept that the odd bad night is not going to kill you, it doesn't mean anything, and is something every normal sleeper experiences from time to time. When you don't care whether you will sleep or not, all pressure is gone and sleep comes effortlessly.

You will only learn to sleep better by not making a fuss when you don't!

These days, if I have a less than brilliant night, I *pay no attention to it*, other than perhaps to get up half an hour earlier the next morning. And *because of this*, I honestly cannot remember the last time I had two sleepless nights in a row, even with chronic jet lag or sleeping in a tent. Between now and being 'cured' you are going to miss dozens and dozens more nights, I promise you that! And, here's the important bit, *you will continue to miss them even after you are cured.* So make a start on changing that reaction, and make the future brighter. I'll go even further in saying this ... until you can miss a night without falling apart, you really haven't cured your insomnia at all.

'I tried positive thinking, really I did. But I couldn't do it.'

Now (like almost everything else I talk about!), making a choice to feel good about a sleepless night is *not* easy at first. The first day you get up after a terrible night and try to be positive, everything is going to sound like a lie, you will still feel anxious and miserable, and it will feel like nothing is working. You will think, 'Sasha doesn't know what she's talking about! How can I be positive when I feel like death?' Now, because this is hard at first, *most people give up*, imagining that nothing is working. But this is a big, big mistake. This is what causes you to loop right back to the start. Probably the biggest mistake people make with the 'positive thinking' side of things is in expecting instant results, and then giving up when they don't get them. I often get comments along the lines of 'I tried thinking positively but it didn't work.' Honestly, sometimes I want to shake people! So what's the alternative? Going back to negative thinking? And how's that been working out for you?!

Positive thinking is for life, not just for Christmas

You can't just 'try' being positive; you need to commit to it. You need to be positive whenever you can remember, even if it doesn't feel like it's working, because ... it *won't* feel like it's working in the early days. *It may well feel like nothing is happening at all*, but *keep at it*. Because if you stick with the alternative, what you have now – negative thinking, you are pretty much *guaranteed* to keep your problem firmly wedged in your life.

Do you think I just woke up one day as a perfect sleeper? Of course I didn't. I had plenty of sleepless nights, negative thoughts, and miserable days. My mood, too, would take a path of all sorts of dips and peaks as I recovered. I knew from the outset that I was on the right track with my general attitude and philosophy, but day to day I didn't always feel 100 per cent positive at all. I still had bad nights and bad days and a few terrible nights and terrible days. But what never left me was the commitment; the commitment to getting over my insomnia for good.

And *this* is how I managed it: after a bad night, or during a bad stretch, I always, always, *always* kept my eye on the prize. I sometimes felt bad, I was sometimes utterly exhausted, but I simply filled my day with distractions and refocused on *waiting for the next little run of good sleep*. I *knew* it would come; it *always* did. So I wasn't at all focused on the little spell of insomnia I was currently experiencing, no matter how terrible it was. Instead, I focused on what was coming next. It was almost like I was 'sitting it out' just waiting for things to pick up again. Thus I never wallowed around wondering what went wrong, or why I couldn't get over my problem. During a good stretch I would be thinking, 'This good stretch is lasting *ages*, I must be getting better.' And when a bad stretch kicked in, I would think, 'That last one was a great stretch of good sleep! I wonder how long until the next one.' But although there seemed to be neither rhyme nor reason to this pattern, I *never* questioned why a bad stretch came along, or what the reasons were, or what I had done wrong, or even what I could do to put it right! I just waited for it to end, *as I knew it would*. And *quite quickly*, the bad stretches became more spread apart and lasted for only a couple of days. And eventually it became only the odd couple of nights here and there, and then the odd night. I would do the same on holiday, or in a strange bed, I would just sit it out and look forward to the next good night. And remember, I didn't even have a book to guide me.

Like I say in *The Effortless Sleep Method,* at some point I knew I was on the right path, but I had no idea how long that path was. I knew recovery was coming, and so should you. The path may end tomorrow, or it might end in a year. But if you don't stay on the path, it may never end at all. Can you see yourself cultivating a similar attitude?

When you are in a good patch, just bask in how good it feels – believe that you are getting better.

And if you are in a bad patch, recognise that *this is absolutely and completely normal* and then just look forward to the next little bit of good sleep. In this way, the bad patches get fewer and further between and the good patches get longer. Stop letting the bad nights and the bad parts of your problem fill your thoughts and take all your focus. Don't give them any space in your head, they don't deserve it.

'But I AM being positive and it's still not working.'

Very often negativity is hard to spot in oneself. It can feel like you are really 'trying' to be positive. You may even work out an affirmation; you may even say it a hundred times a day. But the second you stop, you are back in the doldrums again, fretting, worrying, wondering. For example, if you are someone who continually says, 'I am trying to be positive but ...', 'My sleep is much better but ...', then you are probably not being particularly positive at all. You may even fill your head with negative thoughts *about* the positive thinking! For example, 'I don't think these affirmations are working', 'All this positive thinking I'm doing isn't getting me anywhere', 'I can't see this stuff really working.' These sorts of thoughts usually result in your dropping even bothering with the positive thinking side of things.

Quite often someone will write to me to ask why the Method hasn't worked for them. They will be keeping perfect sleep hygiene but will often still be researching, complaining, trying all sorts of new remedies and putting their insomnia before everything else in their life. If you write to me to tell me the Method isn't working, and then go on to give me a 1000-word account of the history of your problem, how bad it is and how much worse and different it seems from all the others you hear about, and how the positive thinking doesn't work … *then you aren't following the Method at all.*

This little exercise will highlight just how negative your thinking really is. You will find this much harder than you think.

****

Technique: The Two-Week Negativity Fast

I am going to show you how to starve your insomnia to death. For the next two weeks, I want you *never* to complain about your insomnia. I mean it. You are not allowed, for two weeks only, to say anything negative about your sleep, not to yourself or to others. I don't care if you have to lie to your family – this is important, and I'm sure God, your mother and karma will forgive you this one little misdemeanour. If you do inadvertently complain, you have to start the whole two weeks again from scratch. You will find it harder than you think. And this will highlight to yourself just how negative your thinking and talk currently are. *Do it!* You will be amazed at the results.

****

'But it's not realistic to suggest that I can I just be happy all the time.'

I have *never* suggested you pretend to be *happy* all the time. Forcing yourself to feel happy all the time will just cause friction and resistance. I am not happy all the time. I can be a really grumpy cow sometimes. During my recovery I often *felt* bad, exhausted, but the most *negative* thought I had was probably along the lines of 'I wonder how long this bad patch will last.'

The following is often all the positivity you need:

'I feel tired and low today, and that's just fine. I'll just take it nice and easy. I'll be extra kind to myself today, and wait for the next bit of good sleep … it won't be long.'

Can you see that even the decision to be 'okay' with feeling bad for a day is better, and more positive, than beating yourself up, despairing, wondering, fretting, twisting yourself up with questions of why you aren't getting better?

When you *instead*, make that decision, even just to *say*, 'Okay, I haven't slept well, but today I'm going to have the best day I possibly can!' a little dent is made in the old pattern, in the old habit. No matter how much of a lie it sounds, you have weakened the vicious circle, just a tiny bit. Try it. You will find that it gives you an instant feeling of release, of relief.

And you know what I'm going to say next: you need to keep this up, weakening the old pattern and starting to create a new positive one.

So make things *difficult* for your insomnia. If you can look for positive things to say about your sleep, and do your best not to let a bad night get you down, even a *tiny* bit, your insomnia will have a much harder time sticking. Every tiny attempt, even if it feels like nothing has changed, will chip, chip, chip away at that negative habit.

'I've read books on positive thinking before. But I'm a scientist. I don't really know that I believe in all this self-help nonsense.'

In the first book, I recommend that you do daily positive affirmations, writing them down and saying them aloud. For some people, this is apparently such a terrible hardship they would rather continue to suffer with insomnia than admit that something so cosmic and woo-woo could possibly work.

Some bad sleepers would rather keep their insomnia than allow something so 'New Age' and unscientific to help them.

Good sleepers don't care *how* it works, only *that* it works.

'But affirmations just make me feel ridiculous. I mean, you can't really change anything just by stating it's the case. No matter how many times I say "the sky is red" it will always still be blue. No matter how many times I say "I can sleep" it doesn't make it true.'

You know, for most of my life I agreed with you. I had always thought that belief was wholly mysterious. An intangible, inexplicable state of being that was immune to the effects of reason, even in the face of apparent facts. I used this argument against people like Richard Dawkins, who spoke of belief as if it ought to be something that corresponds exactly to the facts (not realising that the 'facts' were only those things *he* believed to be true). I was also influenced by the German philosopher Wittgenstein who argued that belief and faith were not amenable to proof, that those seeking to prove or disprove the existence of God, for example, were playing the wrong language game. I found this whole subject utterly fascinating, mainly because it appeared to me that belief was so elusive, so impossible to define, and so difficult to change. But during my recovery from insomnia, I discovered to both my relief and disappointment, that belief is not mysterious at all. Belief can be changed to whatever you choose.

And I am now going to share a potentially life-changing secret with you.

A belief is just a repeated thought.

I'll just repeat that.

A belief is just a repeated thought.

So, what is the easiest way to change a belief? Just pick a thought and repeat it. That's all there is to it! Is the significance of this already beginning to dawn on you? If you want to have a new and more helpful belief, all you have to do is start thinking it. Thinking it, saying it, repeating it, and acting according to it. Over and over, to yourself, to others, on its own and within the new and positive story that you must now start telling about your sleep. I don't know where this little saying came from, but I try to keep it ringing around in my mind.

You cannot allow yourself the luxury of a negative thought.

So why worry about making sure your thoughts are true, when you could be working on making the truth fit your thoughts?

Some of you will be familiar with my little motto, 'The story you tell about your sleep will come true.' This story telling isn't optional. If you don't start telling a drastically different story, nothing is going to change for you, *ever*. It doesn't matter how many new techniques, pills or cures you try … nothing will significantly change while you are still telling a negative story about sleep. The story you tell has a far stronger effect than anything else you do.

This is why the affirmations are so important. *Yes,* they do sound silly and contrived. But do you have the discipline *always* to remember to keep your sleep talk positive? I doubt it. It is just too easy to fall into negative thinking and speaking. The affirmations provide a disciplined way to make sure that for at least part of the day, your sleep talk is in the right direction.

****

Technique: How to Do Affirmations

So, pick something you would like to be true, the *belief* that you think a really good sleeper would have. *A belief that would allow you to sleep.* For you, it could be 'I'm still a *great* sleeper under all this', 'I trust that I can sleep really well', 'I *can* control my thoughts', I can sleep right through the night.' It can help to start with affirming a belief that is not too far from your current thinking. So, don't start with 'I am the best sleeper in the whole world'; start with 'I seem to be sleeping a lot better these days' or 'I think I am actually getting a bit better.' If you have sleep-maintenance insomnia, try 'I'm sleeping through much better these days.' These can slowly be upped in 'intensity' until you really do believe you are a world-champion sleeper.

If you are very anxious, affirmations can sometimes work to keep you reminded of your problem. In this case, try using less sleep-based ones such as 'I feel so calm/relaxed/centred.' Just the affirmation 'Life is good' or 'I am so happy' can work wonders.

Make sure your affirmation is framed in the positive (no 'nots', no 'don'ts') Stick it on Post-it® notes all over the house, and begin to repeat it *out loud*. When you say it, say it *with feeling*; really feel the meaning of the words. *Just mere repetition is pointless*; you must try to feel it, believe it. Sometimes, put the accent on different parts of the sentence: 'I'm still a *great* sleeper', or 'I'm *still* a great sleeper.' Try saying it to yourself in the mirror – this is really tough but is extra-effective. Say your affirmation(s) about ten times, at least six times a day. You cannot do this too much. A funny thing will very quickly happen: your mind will start looking for things to make it true and focusing on them. Soon, it won't sound like a lie any more, and before you know it *it will be true*. Believe me, *this is how all beliefs are formed – repeated thought.*

Louise L. Hay has based an entire methodology around affirmations and written dozens of books on the subject, including the international bestseller *You Can Heal Your Life*. If you enjoy using affirmations, do look her up.

****

'How does positive thinking actually work?'

It may reassure you scientific types to know that I do *not* currently believe in a mystical 'law of attraction'. Now, I'm not saying there's anything wrong with believing in a law of attraction. But I do not believe there's anything law-like going on. To call what is going on a 'law' is, I believe, to misunderstand the definition of a law. However, I do know there is a very strong *tendency* to get more of what you focus on. And, at least in the case of insomnia, we don't need anything mystical, cosmic, or magical to explain it (although I have absolutely *no* argument with those who do so).

Insomnia is a habit. And there really is nothing mysterious about a habit. I like to view habits in a very similar way to the way I view beliefs: When you have a thought, feeling or experience, synapses fire in the brain in a certain pattern. The more you repeat this same experience, the stronger the brain's tendency to repeat that pattern of firing. And so the more reinforced and stronger becomes that firing. Adding emotion to the pattern just strengthens it further. Eventually, that firing becomes automatic – and we have a fully formed habit (or belief). As far as I know, this is backed up by science, even if I haven't put it in wholly scientific terms.

For argument's sake, let's say there is one basic brain pattern for the belief 'I'm a bad sleeper'. Now, this pattern is triggered by not sleeping. But the same pattern will *also* be fired by such things as:

- saying 'I'm not a good sleeper'
- calling yourself an insomniac
- taking sleeping pills or anything else 'for sleep' (as opposed to reducing the dosage)
- researching cures
- complaining about sleep, and so on.

So as you can see, it is not just sleeping badly that triggers that habitual 'I'm-a-bad-sleeper' pattern. Sleeping badly is just *one* trigger, not the only trigger.

If you are still taking pills, thinking negatively, worrying, researching new cures then these will conspire to fire the old 'I'm a bad sleeper' pattern *even when you do get good sleep*. This explains why a few good nights of sleep do not instantly result in a positive new belief being formed.

All those other triggers, such as complaining about your sleep, researching cures or worrying, are still in place, and are still maintaining that belief.

This means there is very little chance of one or two good nights weakening this negative pattern. The odd good night, or even run of good nights, is often followed by the odd bad night, *because a few good nights of sleep are not usually enough to cancel out all the* other *contributors to the pattern.*

That old negative pattern is *slightly* weakened by a good night but not enough to stop it from firing completely. This also explains why the thinking so often remains rather negative even when the sleep has picked up. So when it comes to a habit, continually focusing on something by thinking about it, worrying about it, trying to work it out, treating it or researching it creates a habitual thought pattern; it reinforces a particular neuronal firing. Forget any law of attraction stuff; this in itself is enough to explain why focusing on insomnia results in more insomnia.

Now, there is only one way to stop a bad habit: you need to stop that brain pattern from firing so often. You can also weaken or even 'cancel out' that pattern, by doing, saying or experiencing the opposite of all these things.

This same mechanism by which insomnia is created can be used to destroy it.

For example: think about tonight. Think about lying in bed unable to sleep. Think about feeling filled with worry, panic … think about how that makes you feel … *right now*. I'm sure it makes you feel terrible. Imagine what this sort of thinking, this sort of feeling, this sort of *focus* does to your beliefs, and to the chances of your actually sleeping tonight.

Okay, now stop that! When you start to see just what you are doing to yourself and your life with thought and focus, you can begin to change everything for the better. If you are focused continually on what you fear most *then more fear is what you will get.* More fear and more of the thing you are fearful of! So, from now on … focus not on what you fear, but on *where you want to go.*

****

Technique: Focusing on the End Result

I am creating all sorts of positive changes in my life these days just by taking my focus *off* what I *don't* want and gently moving it to what I *do* want. Try moving your thoughts to what you *would* like to happen, to where you *want to be.* For me, the focus usually goes to the next day, rather than the night. After all, if the next day is sorted, the night will take care of itself. So, place your focus on tomorrow, on waking feeling good, after a long undisturbed night, relaxed without a spot of anxiety. Or focus on a future time, when you are sleeping normally and all is well. Again, this is hard in the beginning and your mind will doubtless fight and attempt to sabotage things. But keep it up. This little technique gets surprisingly quick results and the sabotaging will then tend to drop away.

****

'I believe what you say in principle, but it seems I have absolutely no control over my thoughts. My negative thinking, fears and worries about sleep are sabotaging everything. It's like there's a really powerful voice at the back of my mind saying, "You know none of this will ever work, you're not going to sleep tonight, there's something wrong with you, and you'll never get better." I can't shut this voice up, no matter how hard I try.'

Yes, you can. You just haven't tried hard enough or for long enough.

If you have a strong active mind, it is likely to jump in at every opportunity to sabotage, put a negative slant on, everything and make you feel powerless and hopeless. I have no idea why the mind does this, but rest assured, it happens to almost all of us. I don't truly understand self-sabotage but I suspect it is down to some misguided strategy for keeping you safe.

I am not trained as a psychologist, so I probably am about to give a fairly unscientific explanation of what I think is going on; nevertheless it seems to work.

There do seem to be two aspects to our thinking and belief. There is the active mind, and then there is a deeper, more mysterious side, in which reside our beliefs, our strongly held beliefs. And it is this deeper side that we need to influence. The problem is, whenever we try to think a new belief, such as 'I can sleep perfectly well unaided', the voice jumps in and says, 'No you can't, you are broken, an insomniac, you're getting worse and you'll never get better.' And it all seems hopeless. If only we could get a few nights' sleep, we think, then perhaps this belief would change … but of course, the belief itself stops us from sleeping, and the whole thing becomes a vicious circle.

Later in the book, I am going to show you how to work directly on those beliefs. Now, the reason I have digressed so much to talk about this self-sabotaging side of your mind is this: *it won't necessarily feel like anything is happening*. But this doesn't mean it isn't. So many people write to me to say, 'I tried affirmations but they didn't work.' Or, 'I did that process you told me about yesterday but it didn't do anything.'

The most important thing to remember is that changing beliefs is like changing a habit; it works by using repetition, repetition, repetition. So just because you feel like nothing is changing, it doesn't mean this is true. Your deeper, unconscious mind is listening, listening, listening *always*. So, even when you 'fake it' and your conscious mind 'laughs at you', your unconscious still hears. At some point, with enough repetition, *the belief will start to change*, the laughing will stop, the sabotage will diminish. *And you will not consciously 'feel' this happening*. You will just realise one day that things seem to feel a bit more positive and everything is somehow a bit easier.

This is going to sound crazy, but the main reason positive thinking is hard is because you *think* it is hard. You find it hard to change your thinking, because you *think* you can't. You think that because that negative voice is still there, that nothing is ever changing, that it will never change. This just isn't true.

'Can you give me something practical to do to help change my negative thoughts and beliefs? Sometimes it just feels like I can't stop the negative thought popping in. Then I feel bad and frustrated.'

Up until now, a lot of what I have said has been theoretical. But now I'm going to give you *two* cast-iron ways of dealing instantly with negative thoughts and achieving a positive change in beliefs.

One problem with having a book chock-full with techniques is that they usually get ignored.

The danger is that you read through, get to a technique, say, 'I'll do that later, I'm enjoying reading right now' and promptly forget all about it. So I ask you now: if you find yourself unable to cope with negative beliefs or troublesome thoughts, you really should come back and try these two little techniques.

The first is what I call the 'Stop Thinking Technique'. Let's go back to my coughing fits to illustrate this, because it is a simpler example than insomnia. In getting over my coughing fits, I remember:

1. I would do my best to relax gently when I felt the feeling of needing to cough, rather than panicking over it. But then, more importantly,

2. I would immediately *move my mind to a different subject.*

Eventually, the connection between meetings and coughing began to weaken. Gradually, I began to break down that connection until my brain gave up firing in that pattern. I'm not sure when, but at some point the pattern became completely broken. Today, I wouldn't even remember to remember to cough in a meeting!

I didn't mention this in *The Effortless Sleep Method* because I didn't deem 'stopping thinking and moving my mind to a different subject' to be an actual technique in its own right. I suppose I imagined that everyone would know to do this. But judging by all the questions I received in relation to negative thoughts, I soon came to realise this was not the case. In fact, by the time I came to finish this book, I was advising almost every new consultation client about this 'Stop Thinking Technique', as I now call it. Don't be fooled by its apparent simplicity. Doing the following may be all you need to do to turn your negative thinking around. *If you use only one technique, use this one.* This is *exactly* how I overcame the coughing problem I mentioned earlier. It also played a *large* part in my overcoming 'special event insomnia'. If you have seemingly uncontrollable obsessive thinking, this will be the ideal technique for you. I have since found out that it is not unlike what NLP (neurolinguistic programming) therapists call 'a pattern break'.

****

Technique: The Stop Thinking Technique

When a negative thought pops into your head, perhaps, 'Oh no, I have an important meeting tomorrow. I'm never going to sleep tonight!' you need to do the following. Gently but immediately, stop thinking the negative thought and start thinking something, *anything* else. Think about ... what to have for lunch, what's on television tonight, that person at work you fancy, that person at work you hate, you must phone your mother, you need to buy some tea bags, the colour of the dog walking outside the window, where you want to go on holiday, the meaning of life, a prayer to God, *anything!* You need to do this *as soon* as a negative thought or fear decides to pop in.

Now, this won't work straight away because the negative thought will carry on trying to show itself and take your attention. Just ignore it and keep thinking of other things. Eventually, one of these thoughts will take your attention, fill your mind and set off a new train of thought. And ... that original negative thought will be forgotten and it grows weaker.

Some people use the same technique, but instead of thinking a different thought, they distract themselves with a physical activity. You could try going for a nice walk, or even something not so nice, like clearing out an old drawer or putting on a load of washing. Every time you do this, that habitual thought pattern becomes weakened, and thus becomes less habitual, less automatic. Do this enough and the brain will give up firing in this way, and the negative thoughts won't occur at all.

According to some schools of thought, blocking or suppressing negative thoughts and feelings is not advisable. So it *may* not be a good idea to use this technique for lifelong issues, such as traumatic memories. But we are not talking about deep-seated, identity-creating issues, we are talking about pointless, troublesome thoughts such as 'If I don't sleep tonight, I'll feel terrible tomorrow.' Moreover, I am not talking about blocking or suppressing. I am talking about moving your mind away from that troublesome thought onto a different subject. Because this thought is a niggling, pointless thought, if you stop giving it attention it will eventually wither and die.

****

'What about the more deep-seated negative beliefs?'

Okay, the second wonderful, life-changing technique you really should perfect is this one.

One thing that can scupper us when trying to install a new belief is the existence of a diametrically opposed negative belief. This can make affirmations less effective and take a lot longer to 'stick'. And I know that if progress is slow, you are likely to give up. So let's work on dissolving those negative beliefs, and we will find, miraculously, that the positive new beliefs will be born automatically.

This is a slightly altered reframing process which I think works much, *much* better than the standard CBT (cognitive–behavioural therapy) reframing. It has been influenced by Byron Katie and her 'four questions to change your life'. I never found Byron Katie's work particularly helpful personally, but after meeting her in London, and hearing the testimonies of so many trusted people, this led me to tweak her questions for my own benefit. If you find the following helpful, do look up Byron Katie herself. She is quite a woman with millions of devoted followers. You may well find her work more helpful than I did.

I feel CBT has missed out the almost 'meditative' quality of this sort of process, concentrating entirely on finding rational, intellectual alternatives to our unhelpful thoughts. If you look at Byron Katie's work, there is no sense of this being an intellectual process at all.

Byron Katie and CBT are using the same process. But CBT does not allude to the 'instinctive, meditative' quality of this process, and Byron Katie's more 'spiritual' version may alienate those with a more scientific, rational bent. Which interpretation do I favour? I am too pragmatic to choose. Both are using the same technique and *that* it works is enough for me; I really don't care *how* it works.

Working on beliefs only feels difficult now because you think that your negative beliefs are part of 'who you are'. They are *not*. A negative belief has nothing to do with who you are. It's just nonsense, a harmful, repeated thought that has served you very badly.

To work on reframing beliefs, you need to do the following. You must, and I repeat, you *must* write all your answers down. This simply doesn't work properly if you try to do the process in your head. And don't try too hard to find a sensible answer.

There are no wrong answers in this process. It is as much about 'feeling' as it is about thinking. It's about just letting thoughts and feelings arise.

****

Technique: The Magic Belief-Changer

1. I want you to identify, and *write down* all of the beliefs you have about your sleep and your problem. You could try asking yourself, 'What belief would allow me to sleep tonight?' What is the belief that is getting in the way of *that* belief being true? Write a whole list of all the beliefs that may be stopping you from sleeping *tonight*.

2. Pick out what you feel to be the two or three 'strongest' beliefs. These are the ones you will work on, one at a time.

3. Now, take the first belief, sit quietly and write down how this belief makes you *feel*.

4. Next write down what is ridiculous about this belief? Find a reason, any reason, that that negative belief isn't true. *Wait for the answers. They will come.* Write it all down.

5. Now, if you don't change this belief, what will it ultimately cost you in terms of your life, sleep, relationships, or happiness? What would be the ultimate outcome if you never changed this belief? *Wait for the answers. They will come.* Write your answers down.

4. Next, I want you to consider how life would be *if you believed the opposite*. Get a feel for that now. How would life be different in terms of relationships, career, happiness, *if* you no longer had this harmful belief. How would it feel *if* it were true, just *if*? Don't start trying to believe it; just imagine how it would feel if you didn't

have that thought ... *Wait for the answers. They will come.* Write your answers down.

5. Finally, you are then going to find a new way, a positive way, of viewing that very same situation. If you have done this process thoroughly enough, you will find that a positive answer comes quite naturally. Write down a new way of seeing this very same situation. You should find that, now, this 'reframe' comes much, *much* more easily. Feel lighter? Feel a sense of relief, of hope even? See what you have done? In trying it on for size, you have got a sense of what it would be like to actually have that belief, and in doing so, you have begun to install that belief. If you don't feel a sense of lightness, try a slightly different way of viewing the issue.

Important: This is *not* about finding rational, intelligent, considered answers to the questions. It is about letting your feelings come up, dissolving the 'stuckness' around certain beliefs.

If you feel no different, and are just as hopeless, or feel a massive resistance to reframing one particular thought or belief, move on to a different one and return at a later time. For some reason, some thoughts are sometimes easier to reframe than others. It can help to be quite *specific*. Rather than working on the very generalised belief such as 'I'm a bad sleeper', in the beginning, try working on such beliefs as 'I'll feel wired and stressed tomorrow if I don't sleep' or 'I'll wake up tomorrow at 4am.' These more 'precise' beliefs are easier to get your teeth into. Plus, you can see the instant, tangible, real-world results of your efforts.

Once you have got the hang of this with one thought or belief, you can move on to every negative belief. With practice, you can even learn to do this 'in the moment' so that a 'bad' thought no longer has any lasting power over you. You will come to see that 90 per cent or more of our thoughts are not 'true' and do not refer accurately to real-life situations. They are simply interpretations, and a negative interpretation is generally no more accurate than a positive one.

And you don't have to restrict this just to the sleep-based beliefs. You can also work on such things as: 'I am always anxious', 'I am different/broken', 'There's no way I'll ever get better'.

When you get the hang of reframing your beliefs, you will want to try it on everything!

This technique can be used as a useful preliminary step before doing affirmations. We all know that in the beginning, affirmations all sound like lies. But if you do this process *first*, you will have the strength of *your beliefs* to back you up. By dissolving strong, opposing negative beliefs, you will find that the wanted, positive affirmations will be able to 'stick' much more easily. That means that these affirmations and safety thoughts won't feel so shaky or untrue. The effect of this can be miraculous and will speed things up exponentially.

****

'But right now, I'm at rock bottom. I can't even imagine how it would feel to be positive. I am desperate and have no hope.'

It may surprise you to hear that most people write to me at the point when they are absolutely desperate; they may well have bought the book, looking for answers, for a magic bullet, for the one amazing piece of advice or technique that will lead them out of their hell. These poor souls use phrases such as:

- I don't know how much more I can take.
- I think I'm going mad.
- I'm reaching breaking point.

- I'm on the edge of the abyss.
- I'm in my own personal hell.

Good news, desperate ones! I've been there too, and have come out the other side unscathed.

It is no wonder that the desperate person cannot sleep. Desperate people are usually unwilling or too unmotivated to follow common-sense instructions. They want something to *make* them sleep *now*. They are looking for someone to give them guaranteed, instant sleep and anything less just isn't appealing to them. Desperate people will usually give the best, most vivid and flamboyant descriptions of how terrible they feel. In other words, they couldn't really be *less* positive about their sleep. They really couldn't be telling a more *negative* story. And this negative story is coming true, again and again.

Please, don't think I am being unsympathetic because I am. But I am not *here* to give sympathy; I am here to help you sleep. Sympathising with your terrible emotional state may make you feel comforted for a few minutes, but won't deal with the problem in hand. So, let's deal with the problem in hand.

'Now, be reasonable', you say. 'How on earth does one who is in this appalling state, in this 'dark night of the soul' *not* feel and speak incredibly negatively?'

The answer is: you don't. You can't. You can't do anything when you are in this state. Of *course*, all you can focus on is sleep, and how much you want it. That is why it is so tempting to take a pill at this time, or to take a nice big cocktail of the damnable things, all washed down with a large whiskey.

The really sad thing is that most people turn to help only when they are feeling at their most desperate. They wait until a really bad night has occurred to make an appointment with a doctor or therapist ... or they email me. I remember doing the same. I would spill my appalling story out to the poor doctor or therapist (making sure they knew in great detail just how terrible was my suffering).

So you go to the doctor and say, 'I just need some sleep', and the doctor gives you something 'to make you sleep'. Or rather, s/he gives you something to make you *unconscious*. (There is a *big* difference and this difference is important.) The horrible irony is, this is very *worst* time to start experimenting with a new technique, pills, method, CD, listening to a new therapist, contacting me etc. Because, the truth is, when you are this desperate, *nothing* will *make* you sleep, no matter what you do or take. Your tension is so high and your belief so low that your body is fighting desperately to keep you awake. All a pill will do now is knock you unconscious until it begins to wear off in the small hours, at which point your body will wake you with an unpleasant start, without your having had anything *like* refreshing sleep.

So, what on earth can we *do* when we feel like this? Well, the fact is that you can't do anything much when you are in this state. I have been there, many, many times. Any relaxation recordings, including the Sleep Tools, are going to be ineffectual right now. And the positive affirmations and visualisations are going to have a tough time sticking when you are in this state.

But this desperate state never lasts.

There always, always comes a better night or day, sooner or later. So try to let this be a comforting thought: *There is nothing to do, nothing to tussle over, nothing to try or test.* Be as a child and stop trying to get it right. Don't look to cures at this point, don't look for something new to try, something to 'do'. Just sit it out, keep the sleep hygiene tight, get on with your life as normally as you can, and wait until the next good night. Have the attitude 'It may be tonight, it may be tomorrow, it may be next week, but it'll come eventually.' With *this* attitude, that good night will be sure to come a lot faster than if you carry on thinking 'I just *have* to sleep tonight, I *must* sleep tonight, I'll *die* if I don't sleep tonight'! Keep up this thinking, and that desperation will push the good night further away. So for now, just relax and stop trying to do anything. Perhaps meditate, go for a walk, watch a film, get exercise: not 'to make you sleep', but just to make you feel a bit nicer. *This horror will pass.* You will get to a better place soon, and it is *only* from this better place, that you can be back in a position of power and start building hope and belief.

So, how do we get to a better place?

Well, in a sense, you need to get a *bit* better before you can get a *lot* better … and *this* is why the sleep hygiene is so important. When your sleep hygiene is really good, and you are taking active steps to relax, sooner or later there *always* comes a better night's sleep. I know it's hard to believe this when you are feeling so low, but sooner or later, there is *always* a better night, maybe two. And this is when the recovery can really start. This is when you can start to celebrate your little success, turn your thoughts to the positive, start really getting into the affirmations, practise the Belief-Changer Technique I describe earlier in this chapter and *stop all negative talk about sleep.* From this new positive place finding good things to think and say will be much easier.

Just to illustrate this, consider the following.

Earlier in this book, I described how I would sometimes ignore emails from those who were demanding that I answer their one vital, key question about insomnia. Completely by accident, I came to use a similar method for dealing with the most desperate, pleading emails. I used to answer all email questions personally and without charging for my time. My email load fast became huge (and eventually unmanageable), which meant that quite often it would take me up to a week or more to get back to people. Some of those people had written to me at 5am, in a state of utter desperation and by the time I eventually wrote to them, it was too late to help them with that immediate problem.

But … I noticed something interesting happening here.

When I eventually replied, these people almost inevitably then said words to the effect of 'Actually, I've been sleeping much better since that night. Sorry for the meltdown.' In fact, this happened *so* often that I started a different tactic – when anyone wrote to me in a really desperate state, I would *intentionally* ignore them, even if I had the time to answer them immediately. I would even fire off a short email, telling them I couldn't answer yet, but to sit tight, help was coming soon. Now, usually this was true, especially in the later days, but sometimes *it wasn't*. It was a tactic of mine.

This little tactic of mine revealed two things:

1. First of all, this 'point of desperation' is not the best time to give advice, take advice, or to do anything much at all. Just like leaving de-stressing activities until bedtime, there's really not much you can do at this point. Your state of mind is not receptive, your negativity is heightened, and you can't even think sensibly.

2. Second, and more importantly, it shows that this one bad night, this one bad stretch, which seems *so* important at the time, is pretty irrelevant in the grand scheme of things.

'But it doesn't feel like I need help when I've been sleeping well for a few nights. That's why I turn to help only when I need it.'

This is a common mistake: if you have been sleeping well for a week or two, somehow it just doesn't feel important or even relevant to be doing 'positive thinking' or even keeping the sleep hygiene good. After a few nights of good sleep, many people just let all the good habits go. Sleep then deteriorates and a few weeks later, they then write to me, desperate again, to ask what has gone wrong.

Letting things go in the good times is one of the worst things you can do (at least in the early days, before a permanent habit has been created). If you let go of the good habits too quickly, it is only a matter of time before a bit of stress or some event comes along to trigger a bad spell. As I explained previously, everything is doubly difficult when you are in the middle of a bad patch and are feeling anxious or depressed.

Instead, also use the *good* times to do something about your insomnia – because it is so, *so* much easier to do and say positive things when you are already feeling good and positive! In doing this you can, relatively effortlessly, increase your general, overall positivity levels. When sleep is good, you should be using this time to springboard your recovery. When you are already feeling positive, affirmations and positive thinking in general have a much easier time sticking.

'I'm doing well at the moment, but I am still terrified about the prospect of another bad patch of sleep. Things feel so good now and I just couldn't bear it all going wrong again. What can I do to shake off this persistent fear?'

If you wait until a high-pressure night looms, or a missed night comes, you obviously have less chance of coping well. So, instead of dreading that day and then panicking when it arrives, use the good times to prepare *now* for that sleepless night when and if it occurs. That way, when a bad night comes, or a high-pressure night looms, you won't even *need* to work on changing your thoughts.

Prepare in advance for a possible missed night by being as positive and upbeat as possible. Do your best to avoid dreading and fearing the next bad night. Instead, attempt to think dispassionately about the possibility of a missed night, rationally, sensibly. Think about how well you will be able to cope with it now. Remind yourself that bad nights always come to an end. Remind yourself that you are getting better now. Remind yourself that everyone misses a night here and there. Remind yourself that missing a bad night is really not a big deal. When you are better prepared, those bad nights will have less of an impact, and one missed night would be just that – one missed night.

This does not mean *expecting* to miss sleep. Rather, we are trying to cultivate a state of 'take it or leave it'. You fully expect and hope it will be a sunny day tomorrow, but if it rains, you don't go to pieces. It's the same with insomnia. You fully hope and expect to sleep like an angel tonight, but if you don't, you'll get on with your day as best you can. Or better still, you will use that opportunity to show just how brilliant a day you can still have.

Often I would challenge myself to have the best day I possibly could after a sleepless night. This is a very powerful thing to do, because it really is showing courage instead of fear in the face of sleeplessness. And when you don't fear insomnia, insomnia becomes powerless.

'I have been making really excellent progress and my sleep is miles better. But I am still having various problems.'

Once you have seen some real progress, it can be irritating that so many little issues take so long to drop away. Your sleep is good, but there are still so many small imperfections that seem not to disappear. Perhaps you are sleeping better but it's still taking you far longer than you would like to fall asleep at night. Or, while your thoughts are mainly positive, sometimes the annoying fear pops in that 'it could all come back'.

I now want to talk to you about a strange phenomenon.

It is very, very common for insomniacs to have an inaccurate view of their own problem. It's a funny thing, but we insomniacs often have a distorted idea about our own success. We start to improve, but instead of focusing on those great nights, we seem only to see the bad ones, even when the good ones are increasing or are even outweighing the bad. It's like the anxiety, stress and fear surrounding insomnia doesn't 'heal' as fast as the sleep itself, so even when the sleep has improved, the thoughts, beliefs and fears remain where they were.

Sometimes, when we are overcoming insomnia, it's almost like we can't see the wood for the trees. When we look too closely, examining every tiny nuance of our sleep, our lack of sleep, and everything else in between, this distorts our view of the situation. I want you to know that I once made the *very* same mistake. Once I started to recover, I still had a totally distorted view of how bad my sleep really was. Yes, I was miles better, but … and there was always a 'but', and that 'but' always got all the attention.

'Are you trying to tell me that my sleep is actually better than I think it is?'

That is certainly possible. I have heard 'insomnia stories' every day for around seven years now, and one thing I notice is that there is no direct relationship between the lack of sleep a person gets and their reaction to it. Those who regularly miss entire nights are not always those who are the most worried. On the other hand, I often get an email like the following:

> I feel like I'm going mad, please help me, you're my only hope, I don't think I can stand any more. I used to get eight hours every night, now I only get seven! And this has been going on for almost three weeks!

Such a person getting 'only' seven hours would probably end up feeling suicidal after missing a whole night, whereas some of the more serious clients would give their right arm to be able to sleep seven hours per night; they would consider this totally 'cured'.

A lack of awareness of the progress they have made is often one of the key things that stop people from making a *full* recovery. And it leads people to write to me, saying things like:

- 'Overall: good. But last night ...'

- 'I've been sleeping like an angel, but some nights it's still taking me two hours ...'

- 'I was med-free for four weeks, but then last night I couldn't resist ...'

- 'I now sleep perfectly in the spare room, but not in my own bed ...'

- 'I'm sleeping well and feeling generally good, but I still can't sleep through the night without waking ...'.

All they can see is failure. All I can see is success. All I want to hear is the 'med-free', the 'sleeping like an angel', the 'overall good'. *This* is where you need to be focusing. Instead of immediately looking to what is still imperfect. You need to learn to recognise every little bit of progress. You need to focus on success *and only success*, wallow in it, exaggerate it! For example, if a bad night comes along out of the blue, try thinking, 'Wow! It's been *ages* between this and my last bad night. I can't *wait* for the next good stretch!'

Remember, this is not about accepting the status quo. Acceptance does not mean stagnation. Focusing on those good nights will result in more good nights. Focusing on what is still bad will only result in more bad.

Do you want to know the best thing to do about niggling remaining issues?

Do nothing. Nothing at all.

Instead of focusing directly on doing something about those problems, at this point it is much more effective to focus on *where you want to go*. Focus on what you *want* to happen, not on what to do about what you *don't* want to happen! (You may need to read that twice.)

And if you are at the stage of only having niggling last issues, I think it's time for you to move on to the final step in overcoming insomnia.

A quick summary of the main positive thinking points:

1. It won't feel like it's working but this doesn't mean it isn't.

2. Prepare to miss more nights, rather than doing all you can do avoid them.

3. Getting better is as much about coping with the bad nights as it is about getting good sleep.

4. Thinking positively is a full-time job.

5. Don't waste time trying to work out what you did wrong when you miss a night (unless it is quite obvious).

6. Remember that bad times *always* come to an end.

7. Ignore the saboteur.

8. It takes time; recovery doesn't happen overnight *ever*.

9. You should be spending very little time thinking about your problem. If thinking about the problem shows itself, you should distract yourself or move your mind immediately to another subject.

10. Use the good times to boost your success; don't let it all go once you start sleeping better.

11. You may not be the best judge of your own problem or success.

ୡଠ

Stage Four
Being
Not a Good, But a *Great*, Sleeper ...

I had considered calling this section 'Advanced Effortless Sleep', because the following advice is not to be taken lightly and it is not recommended that those just starting out should attempt to follow it. This is a densely written chapter and you may need to read it through several times to fully understand the principles I am trying to get through to you. However, the speed of your *complete* recovery will depend entirely on how quickly you can implement the advice in this chapter.

> *'I've settled into a nice routine with the Method. I hardly ever miss a night and when I do I can cope quite well. But I still spend a lot of time thinking about sleep. I just want to put this behind me and go back to the way I was.*
> *Sasha, be honest, will I ever be "normal" again?'*

This final stage is all about how to move past the whole sorry memory of insomnia. At some point, you need to take the final step towards *being* a great sleeper, not just an 'okay' sleeper. Not 'much better' but 'completely better'. Not a 'recovering insomniac' but an 'ex-insomniac'.

One thing that makes insomnia such an especially difficult habit to break permanently is that it pervades one's entire life. You may feel the effect of it constantly, every second of the day and night. When a problem has gone on for many years, the sufferer has usually unwittingly created an entire life, an entire identity around the insomnia. We could say that your *identity* is as *an insomniac.* What's more, you have a whole bank of memories ready to jump in and remind you of this, and a whole host of experiences to prove it. That identity then begins to shape and to dictate how you live every part of your life, what you do, what you think, what you believe, how you act.

Now, great improvements can occur; you can have stretches of really good sleep; but the problem never really leaves you. It's still lurking somewhere, hiding at the back of your mind. And so, sooner or later, the problem returns. It's almost like a voice says, 'That's enough, you can't get any better than this; you are an insomniac, remember? You don't *really* get better, remember? Things only work for a short time, remember?'

And so a bad night comes along, often just when you thought you had really turned a corner. The identity is reinforced, the voice is proved right, the progress is halted and you become despondent. And the pattern repeats, and repeats, and repeats.

Your identity, your belief that you are essentially a bad sleeper just won't allow major, permanent improvement to happen. It continually seeks reinforcement and validation for your current belief, and it achieves this by stopping you from sleeping. This is one reason that sleep aids, pills and remedies are usually completely ineffectual for very long-term problems. The insomniac identity is just too strong to allow any major change. It bemuses me that doctors haven't cottoned on to this, but instead continue to prescribe drugs to long-term sufferers.

Perhaps, slowly over time, as your sleep improves, this identity will begin to change on its own. Sadly, my experience tells me that this long slow improvement isn't actually what happens. Most people reach a certain level of improvement, and then become 'stuck'. Their sleep improves massively, but it still fills a lot of their thoughts. They still have trouble with strange beds, hotel rooms, special events. They become 'okay' sleepers but the problem doesn't ever really leave them.

So how do we move beyond? How do we get to a stage where we are no longer 'a recovering insomniac', but rather 'an ex-insomniac'?

It takes direct, conscious, positive action to change the thinking, to break down this belief and create a new one. Otherwise this pattern will continue to repeat, no matter what you otherwise do, take or try. The only way to tackle a problem like this is by undermining its very foundations.

A Little Background Philosophy

My entire method is underpinned by 15 years of crippling insomnia, followed by my recovery, further research to formalise this knowledge into a cure, and then two years of sleep therapy consultations, where I got to hear all the questions that were still bothering people.

However, there is even more to it than that.

In my own search for a cure, I read pretty much every self-help book out there. These books probably saved my life. But until I wrote *The Effortless Sleep Method,* there seemed few really good self-help books written specifically about insomnia.

As a result of my self-help addiction, I came up with my own little set of mottos, partly as a result of my own thinking and insights, and partly distilled from all the best wisdom out there, as I saw it. The philosophy that follows is a kind of précis, a 'meta' method, an explanation of the way I see things working in terms of mind, and experience of the world. When I learned how to cure my insomnia, I didn't just improve my sleep. I improved my whole life. I did this by coming to see that the underlying principles of *The Effortless Sleep Method* can be applied to everyday life.

There was a period of time when I would have the following initials drawn on the back of my hand at all times

ETB   LEBO   BIO

Anyone who knew me at the time will remember the felt-tip scrawlings that always adorned my left hand. Anyway, these stand for:

1. Expect the best.

2. Let everything be 'okay'.

3. Bring it on!

These three attitudes tend to feed each other, so that we end up with the following positive circle of thinking.

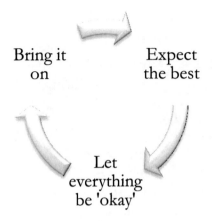

Bring it on → Expect the best

Let everything be 'okay'

The Positive Circle of Thinking

This was the *general* attitude I cultivated in getting over my insomnia and it is how I try to continue to live my life now. I do my utmost to ensure I remain living in this circle. It's quite amazing how my life seems to lift and become freer whenever I remind myself of these words. *The Effortless Sleep Method* encompasses these mottos in the following way:

1. Focus on all the good in your life now, on how good your sleep is and where you want to go, *never* on what is wrong. In other words, *Expect the best.*

2. Take bad nights completely in your stride and don't waste a second's thought worrying about them. In other words, *Let everything be okay.*

3. And finally, grasp life by the horns, go for it, and stop compromising your life for insomnia. In other words, *Bring it on!*

Thus the circle maps perfectly onto the following three fundamental lessons of *The Effortless Sleep Method.*

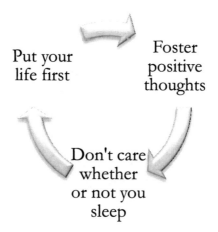

The Effortless Sleep Circle

That's it, really. If you could truly live your life by those mottos (with just a *little* help from good sleep hygiene) you would have no more insomnia. If you, we, all of us, could learn to live our lives by these mottos, it would change the quality of our experience in profound and mind-blowing ways. You may think you already have an attitude to life which is along these lines. Many of us think of ourselves as quite positive people, and imagine that we already think in this way. But my experience of dealing with insomniacs reveals a different picture; the opposite, in fact. I have found that most insomniacs:

- focus on all the things that could go wrong with their sleep

- stress terribly when they do

- compromise their lives by hiding away from all that scares them or could affect sleep.

These three actions then tend to feed each other so that we instead end up stuck in the following negative feedback loop.

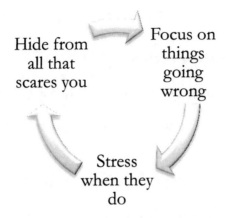

Hide from all that scares you

Focus on things going wrong

Stress when they do

The Negative Circle of Sleep

Now, if you are finding it hard to move on, if you feel you have become 'stuck' in your progress, you are almost certainly living in this third, negative circle.

Although you have made initial progress, you are probably still giving far too much attention to the negative aspects of your sleep; you may be reacting badly to a less-than-perfect night, perhaps wondering and fretting about why they are still happening. And you are very likely still to be making lots of compromises in your life 'because you have insomnia'.

The way out of this vicious circular pattern, to break out of the insomniac identity, is to do nothing less than to *reinvent* yourself *... as a good sleeper!*

And the way to reinvent yourself as a good sleeper is to take a big, bold step into the positive circle and stay there. I know this is difficult, almost impossible at first. But every time you go round the circle, it gets stronger. And the effect is cumulative. You only have to go around a few times to see results ... and you're away.

What you need to realise is that if you really want to be completely insomnia-free, commitment to acting according to/living in the positive circle is not *optional*.

1. You *must* focus on the success, when it happens,

2. You *must* not panic and go to pieces when you miss a night,

3. And you *must* stop compromising your life for insomnia.

If you don't expect the best, be okay with the outcome and put your life before your insomnia, you will never, and I repeat, never fully get over your problem.

And here's how you do it:

Expecting the Best

From now on, no matter where you are, or how bad your sleep is, you need to *expect the best*. Now, this does not mean 'getting over my insomnia', it does not mean 'sleeping five hours a night', it does not mean 'getting off pills' although all of these are great and worthy stages along the way.

No, I want you to expect the best, the *very best*. I want you to expect to become a *great* sleeper, a *champion* sleeper, an *inevitable* sleeper. *Choose* the outcome you would like to experience. I know that at the moment this seems like an impossibility, ridiculous even. But stay with me; there is light behind the lunacy.

First, simply by raising your expectations by several notches, you will already be focusing on a higher goal, expecting good things, probably way better than you currently are doing and this alone will have a positive effect on your thoughts and attitudes.

But there is a different reason that aiming *so* high is important specifically to insomnia. If you focus on a really magnificent future goal, *it takes the pressure off the immediate details*. The more outrageous the expectation the less idea you will have about how you're going to get there. This means that you can be freer and easier with those specific, irritating little aspects of your problem that can steal your attention and drain you of positivity.

Yes, you'll 'do' things to improve your sleep. But if you're aiming at becoming a really *great* sleeper, the details of sleeping on this or that particular night or 'how to get over this one irritating little thing' *don't really matter*.

Let's look at an analogy: suppose Richard Branson decides that his goal for next year is to make £100m; that is his goal. (I'm sure he doesn't set arbitrary monetary goals like this, but this is just for the purposes of making a point!) Now, having set this goal, he is unlikely, therefore, to fret about the £70 parking ticket he has just received, or the fact that his gas bill has been over-estimated.

In the same way, if you have a goal to become a brilliant, inspirational sleeper, you will be less bothered by a single missed night, or a wayward negative thought, by whether you should have done an extra half hour at the gym, or whether you drank one coffee too many.

Hence the focus is taken *off* what you do, *this second*, lying awake in bed. It is taken *off* what you are going to *do* to make yourself sleep *tonight*. Because, in the grand scheme of becoming a champion sleeper, tonight, this moment, this feeling, this little aspect of your problem, is irrelevant.

These things will seem trivial, will bother you less and so, you will naturally begin to lighten up, to let go of the obsessing.

'But, if I aim that high I'll just be extra disappointed when I fail. Wouldn't it be better to keep my expectations at a modest level, so at least I have a chance of achieving them?'

Yes, that's fine ... if you are happy settling for a mediocre life.

When you live in The Positive Circle, there is no such thing as serious disappointment. Remember: *you let everything be 'okay'.* When you live your life in The Positive Circle, stuff still happens, but there is literally no such thing as failure.

Besides this, I believe the relationship between expectation and disappointment is this:

Aim for the rooftops and you might reach the streetlight.
But you may only get as far as the gutter.

Aim for the moon and you might reach the moon.
But you'll get at least as far as the streetlight.

I sometimes still hear from those who followed my Method years ago, right at the beginning before I had even written the book. A few of them are now teaching others how to sleep better! From chronic insomnia to sleep guru! Do you fancy that role? After all, if you set a goal to become a sleep guru, you might miss your target, but you'll get at least as far as becoming a truly excellent sleeper.

Letting Everything Be Okay

Let's speed things up a bit. If you really want to turbo-charge your recovery, you should take the advice in this section very seriously. In doing so you will really put this insomnia business behind you very quickly indeed.

The *only* way you will know you have been really successful is when, at some future point, you'll look back and realise that you haven't even thought about your sleep problem lately, that you didn't even remember to fuss about sleeping on a high-pressure night, that you couldn't even stay awake for an hour in bed if you wanted to. In fact, you really won't have fully recovered until you have resigned insomnia to history – as some problem you once had.

'I'm ready to really put this behind me. I only have the last remaining niggles to overcome. How best to do this?'

This next point is very, *very* important. The only way to 'put this to bed' for good (excuse the pun) is to forget about it, *really* forget about it. But this point *will never come* if you keep fussing about last 'loose ends', about why you can't move on, about what is *still* wrong with your sleep. How can you possibly forget about insomnia if you remain worried about how long your recovery is taking? And please note that if you have 'last niggling loose ends', this means, by deduction, that the rest of your sleep is pretty good, perhaps even great on occasions. So why are you paying any attention whatsoever to what is wrong, why are you focused on what you *don't want*?

You need to let everything, and I mean *everything* be 'okay'. Be okay with your sleep, however it is, however much you get or don't get – it's just fine. It's 'okay'. So, paradoxical though it may seem, I want you to *pay no attention* to all those things that are still wrong. By trying to sort out 'these last loose ends', *there will always be last loose ends.* By trying to sort out all that is still wrong with your sleep, *there will remain something wrong with your sleep.* While you are still focused on these remaining bits of your problem, *you will still have a problem.*

So, do you want to hear the best advice for what to do about tying up loose ends?

Do nothing. Nothing at all.

So don't write to me to tell me you want advice about tying up the last loose ends. Instead, I want you to ignore the bad times, and 'big up' the good times to the extent that you are almost 'in denial' about the existence of any remaining problems.

'Please, please, please … just one question before I do this! I have just this ONE issue with [insert your issue here] which means I can't make this final step. I have had a few nights when I slept fine anyway, but most of the time this is still a problem.'

No it's not. You don't have a problem. I mean it. You just told me you slept fine a few times despite this issue. You slept fine. *End of story.*

Does this sound like I'm belittling your problem? I'm not. But I *am* trying to make it little. I'm trying to make it go away. Because it's this focusing on what is still bad that is responsible for there still being a problem at all.

This goes for all those things like sleeping in hotel beds, sleeping at a friend's house, sleeping before events, sleeping when you are on your period, sleeping in the summer/winter/when it's raining, sleeping with a new partner, organising parties, and any other remaining issue, niggle or remaining problem. You need to let *everything* be okay.

I want you to focus on the good, *while completely, wilfully ignoring the bad*. From now on 'you sleep great'. Full stop.

If a bad night comes along, it's the fault of the sheets, or the air conditioning, or the neighbours, or some funny food you ate, or *anything*, or *nothing at all*. But it is *never, ever* because 'you can't sleep because of this last remaining issue'. It is never, ever because 'you have insomnia'. It is never, ever because 'you have last niggling problems with sleep'. Because you are a brilliant sleeper, a great sleeper, you sleep better than anyone – *this* is your identity now, let it dictate what you do and say, and the way you see the world. Let's start thinking like a perfect sleeper. What would a perfect sleeper think? What would he or she do?

Let me make an analogy. Think of the way in which a doting mother can only see the good in her child. We all know mothers like this (and I'm sure I'm one of them). A child can be selfish, or very lazy or behave like a little monster. But the child's mother would simply say her child is wonderfully driven, too independent to help anyone else out, and any bad behaviour is a result of lack of stimulation because the child is too intelligent. And so, her child remains perfect in her eyes.

Can you adopt a similar attitude to your sleep? Whatever happens, report it as positively as possible, *even if you have to fake it a bit!* When someone asks whether you are tired, say, 'I'm not too bad, I slept well last night.' Or you could even say, 'I didn't sleep that well because I was too cold. I'll use an extra blanket tonight and sleep like a baby.'

If sleep really doesn't come at all, then either ignore it or blame it on something else. Blame it on *anything* other than your long-standing insomnia problem. Blame it on the Moon in Sagittarius, on fact that the dinner gave you indigestion, or anything, or *nothing*.

Because, that problem is in the past now. You need to bury it, really bury it. You are now 'someone who sleeps night after night'. So there *must* be another explanation for why it didn't happen this time. And then let it go completely, forget it, don't give it another moment's attention, and get on with your day. This is exactly the way a normal good sleeper would act. This is the way you must now act.

Try to foster this attitude in all areas of your sleep. Just like the doting mother and her perfect children: the children can't be selfish, because they're perfect in her eyes. No, they are just very independent. When you don't sleep, it can't be your fault, because you are a perfect sleeper. No, it's the fault of something else.

Bringing It On

And finally, it's time to plunge headlong into the good sleeper identity. Earlier in the book, I described the way that habits are formed. I showed you that not sleeping itself is just one contributor to insomnia. There were also such things as thoughts, certain behaviours and actions all playing their part in maintaining this habit of poor sleep.

Just as there are many different contributors to a habit, this is also true of identity. Every time you allow sleep to affect what you do, think or say, you reinforce the old insomniac identity. Similarly, a perfect sleeper almost inevitably *sleeps perfectly*. But this is really only one small part of the complete picture. There are all sorts of other behaviours associated with being a perfect sleeper. A normal good sleeper goes through life, taking action, making decisions, without even thinking about sleep, and this is where we want to end up.

It's no good sitting waiting for the sleep to pick up, hoping for a slow eventual identity change, because we could be waiting forever. We need to work, *right now*, on forcing the good sleeper identity into existence. And rather than working directly on the sleep, and expecting the identity to follow suit, we can instead can do all those *other* things a good sleeper would do, breaking down the insomniac identity from all directions … and let the *sleep* follow suit.

Your attitude to life, events, risks is *Bring it on.* From now on, there can be no avoidance behaviour whatsoever. There are no more compromises. But you don't just take what life throws at you; you grasp life with both hands and take it for yourself.

Instead of avoiding all those things a good sleeper is able to do, you actively need to start doing them. At some point you need to make plans, see your friends, stay out late, read in bed, book holidays, get back into the world, and start living, thinking, speaking, acting as a good sleeper would act, *and let the sleep come following after you.*

Some of you may have noticed a contradiction in my writing. On the one hand, I am telling you to make no compromises whatsoever for the sake of insomnia. But I also give you a whole list of promises you must make, some of which (such as not reading in bed and getting up early at weekends) could certainly be viewed as compromises. Eventually, we must take steps to normalise your actions surrounding sleep. This means giving up all those compromises we are currently making to the problem, *and this includes some of the promises I ask you to make.* Bizarre as it may sound, at some point in the future, when you are ready, you need to *let go* a little on following my advice.

I don't know if you have read any philosophy, but I want you to consider this quotation from my favourite philosopher, Ludwig Wittgenstein:

> "My propositions serve as elucidations in the following way: anyone who understands me eventually recognises them as nonsensical, when he has used them – as steps – to climb up beyond them. (He must, so to speak, throw away the ladder after he has climbed up it.)
>
> He must transcend these propositions, and then he will see the world aright."

The ladder analogy is absolutely pertinent here. At some point, having used the rules, we must throw them away; we must *forget*. To move *beyond* insomnia, we need to get away from all self-consciousness about sleep. We must move away from 'religious rule following' because the rule following has become a problem in itself. We must *move on*.

Having climbed up, you must now take the leap of faith. You must throw away the ladder.

Become someone who makes big plans, someone with an active social life, who stays out late, lies in sometimes at weekends, reads in bed if they want, and just *lives* like a completely normal person. *This doesn't mean deliberately and artificially breaking the promises;* it means acting just as a normal sleeper would act, like someone who has never had a sleep problem.

'But isn't there a huge danger I'll suffer a massive relapse
if I do too much too soon?'

You may be jumping the gun here. Perhaps this is all a bit quick for you. This sudden move *will* probably cause some missed nights in the early days, and this could lead to despondency. Some of these things – for example, making plans or staying out late – could disturb your sleep in the short term, and you have to feel able to plough on regardless. If you are likely to fall to pieces when that happens, then you aren't ready to take this step. If this holds a huge fear for you, then it's probably too soon to attempt to reinvent yourself as a good sleeper all in one fell swoop.

But don't worry, you can also take little baby steps using the following exercise.

The Acting-As-If Exercise

Put aside some time for the initial preparation. I call this *acting-as-if* because you are going to start acting as if you were a normal good sleeper.

Get a sheet of paper and make a list of as many things as you can think of that a good sleeper would be likely to do or say. Make sure some of these are things you would have avoided because of insomnia. And make some of them are things you wouldn't *dream* of doing because of insomnia.

Next, place them in order of scariness from not particularly scary to really impossible.

Each day, you are going to pick at *least* one thing from the list and *do* it.

You can go as fast as you like, but after one month *or sooner* you need to be doing the slightly scary things.

And after two months *or sooner* you need to be attempting the *really* scary things.

As I said, go as fast as you like, doing as many of these things as you like each day, and repeating them as often as you like. But don't terrify yourself too quickly so that you give up.

So what are some of the things that you could put on your list? Well, these *will* have to be personal to you. Whatever it is that you have stopped doing because of insomnia, the things *you* think a great sleeper would do or say. But here are a few thoughts to get you started:

- Making an appointment to see the doctor about giving up sleeping pills
- Planning a family dinner
- Planning a social event for your friends
- Starting to look for a new job
- Organising a mid-week evening activity
- Reading in bed
- Trying to get pregnant
- Deciding to go just one day without sleeping pills
- Deciding to go just one week without any sleeping pills
- Throwing away all of your remedies, taking your CDs and books to the charity shop
- Book a night in a nice hotel, just for you
- Book a night in a nice hotel, for you and your partner
- Go camping or sleep on the beach

- Watch a midnight cinema showing of a film
- Book the early morning flight, rather than the evening one
- Get up an hour earlier than you need to and watch the sun come up/go for a walk, *just for fun.*

One thing you might consider writing on your list is to throw out all your insomnia-related paraphernalia. You know: the stuff that doesn't work and never has worked? I remember at one point I had a mass clear-out. I threw away all the pills, tapes, masks and even all the books I had ever read in my fight against insomnia. I went through my bedroom and through my cupboards, searching for *anything* insomnia related. If I had bought it because of insomnia, out it went. That was a real key point in my recovery, and is the really empowering type of act you can do when you feel strong enough.

If you start really small, even those at the beginning of their recovery can join in with this exercise. You could decide to drop into the conversation, 'I slept *so* well last night' or 'I slept *so* deeply I couldn't get out of bed this morning' and just leave it at that. If it makes you feel a bit scared and uncomfortable – *good.* That means your mind will no longer seek safety in *not* doing it, and so it will stop being scary.

Then move on, perhaps just *making the appointment* to see the doctor about stopping sleeping pills. If it makes you feel a bit scared and uncomfortable – *good.* That means your mind will no longer seek safety in *not* doing it, and so it will stop being scary.

Then get a bit braver, perhaps make a plan mid-week to see someone socially. If it makes you feel a bit scared and uncomfortable – *good.* That means your mind will no longer seek safety in *not* doing it, and *this* will stop being scary.

Eventually, make a BIG plan – a party or a holiday or something that strikes real fear into your insomniac brain. If it makes you feel a bit scared and uncomfortable – *fantastic.* Because when your mind no longer finds safety in avoiding the *really* scary things, no longer seeks safety in *not* doing them, *it will give up stopping you from sleeping because of them.*

You need to realise that these acts *need* to feel a bit scary at first. If they didn't feel scary then you would simply be acting according to your old beliefs. Without change in the form of these little acts of faith, there can be no new beliefs, no new identity and you'll be stuck where you are now.

And here's the *vital* thing to remember: when you start moving into the scary things: you must take no notice of the effect these things have on your sleep. *Remember to let everything be okay.* Sleep itself is not the important thing here, *belief* is. Each little acting-as-if adds to your new positive belief, strengthening it, *whether or not it helps you sleep on that particular night.* An acting-as-if is *always* a good thing, even if it messes with your sleep one time. Because *next* time, or the time after that, it *won't* mess with your sleep. Then your shiny new belief is born.

So every day, try to do at least one thing that is something that a really good sleeper does. If it feels uncomfortable and untrue, good. That's how it should feel. If it felt okay, nothing would be changing. And all those things that bad sleepers do, complaining about sleep, putting insomnia first, compromising your life – they all need to go out of the window. We need to start you acting-as-if you were a great sleeper. Faking it will soon become making it. And once you have been through a fair few of the items on your list without any problems, *throw the list away.*

'I'd love to be able to take this step of reinventing myself. But I still find it hard to sleep before important occasions. I can't become a really good sleeper until I overcome this.'

I have left the issue of 'special event insomnia' until the very end of this chapter. To some extent, it should be viewed as another 'last niggling problem' – something to be ignored, neglected, forgotten about. But for so many people, it is this issue alone – their reaction to 'special events' – that keeps the insomniac identity strong. It is this very issue that leads so many to begin avoiding events that may affect sleep, and so to avoid life. Special event insomnia is thus intricately tied up with making compromises for sleep. In light of this, I have decided to speak about this at length, to give you detailed, specific advice for overcoming this particularly pernicious problem.

This was the part of my own problem which seemed to linger, even after the rest of my sleep had massively improved. I often felt like I was doomed to lead a boring, flat life. When I had nothing interesting to do, I slept great. But as soon as something fun came along, I wouldn't sleep, ruining my chances of enjoying myself.

Doctors, therapists and family members were always quick to pounce on this, diagnosing it with an overly psychological cause – 'You are clearly punishing yourself, perhaps you unconsciously think you don't deserve to have fun.' 'This is all because when you were a child you lived too far away from your friends.' 'This is because your father died when you were a child and you are too afraid to have fun again in case someone else dies.'

Seriously, what a load of tosh!

The reason why you cannot sleep before important events is simply because of the heightened state of anticipation or excitement that occurs when you are looking forward to, or are apprehensive about, a future event. Eventually, this becomes habitual and the anticipation of a missed night is what keeps you awake, more than the event itself.

If you are anything like me, this will be the last part of your problem to disappear. So, if you are reading this and are still at an early stage, just forget about those high-pressure nights for now. Save working on this problem until you have already improved enough to be taking the leap of faith towards being a great sleeper. Don't try to climb Mount Everest before you have even practised on a hill. In the early stages of recovery you won't yet have strong enough sleep to allow yourself to sleep on these difficult nights. Get to the point where your sleeping is great on 'normal' nights. Keep this up and eventually, this confidence will start to spill over into those high-pressure nights. You will find that as your sleep improves, those events that once intimidated you will slowly drop away and cease to be such an issue. That way, a high-pressure night will sometimes come along and you won't even remember to worry about sleep.

Having said that, there are a few things we can actively do to speed things up.

One reason that these nights can remain so troublesome is because we usually have been unwittingly marking them out as 'special' or different for years. These are the nights when we try something new. These are the nights when we pay extra attention to the time we go to bed. These are the nights when we do our best to make sure every tiny detail, every condition of our going to bed is absolutely and utterly perfect. In other words, we act nothing like a normal good sleeper.

So, first of all, *never* try to do something different or particular on those *individual* 'special' nights, because this is counterproductive. It simply marks them out as 'special' and 'different'. So, if a big high-pressure night is looming, for goodness' sake, don't wait until that night to start using a new technique, or try a new relaxation CD. This will only serve to reinforce the problem.

If you feel very nervous about a future event, there are some things you can do in preparation. One of the very best preparations is to do a little visualisation.

Your brain cannot tell the difference between something you vividly imagine and something you actually experience. Don't believe it? Then try this little experiment: imagine in great detail something really horrific, perhaps a dog being tortured or an old man being mugged at gunpoint. Imagine their terror, imagine their cries …

How did it make you feel? Did it make you feel uncomfortable, did your heart beat faster? Perhaps you found it too distressing even to attempt the visualisation. Did you think me sick for suggesting such a thing? Why? The old man doesn't exist; neither does the dog. So what are you getting upset about?

Of course, the reason you feel stressed is that your body responds as if this event were really happening before your very eyes. The great thing is that this doesn't just work with upsetting thoughts; it works when you imagine lovely, delicious, delightful things too.

You know all those unpleasant memories of sleepless nights and miserable days that you think have so much power over you, the ones you think are stopping you from ever moving on? Wouldn't it be great if we could instead fill your head with new memories, memories of great sleep, of waking up happy and refreshed. It's perfectly in your power to do just that … right now … *before the sleep even picks up*. In fact, you can add a memory right now. You see, there are two ways to create a 'memory': you can actually have that experience in the real world, of deep delicious sleep, *or* you can fake it. And by faking it, you can install any memory you want!

The following is a very simple visualisation exercise that only takes a few minutes. You should consider doing this every day. Some people have a problem conjuring up images, but that's fine. Because what I want you to do is to visualise, or 'rehearse', *feelings*.

****

Technique: The Six-Minute Visualisation

Go to a quiet place where you can be on your own for six minutes. I always feel five minutes is too short a time, and ten minutes is long enough that you might end up making excuses and not doing it. But *everyone* has six spare minutes. You could even do this in the toilet! But it's great to do this in the morning not long after getting up. It is helpful to set an alarm on your phone or watch to go off in six or seven minutes' time. That way you won't be distracted by checking the clock.

Now, take a nice deep breath, close your eyes if you want and begin to imagine you have just woken up, got out of bed, and sat down exactly where you are now, from *the* most *de-licious*, natural, un-drugged sleep you have ever had. The most important thing is that you try to feel the feelings you would feel if you were a perfect sleeper. Imagine yourself feeling refreshed, floppy and relaxed. You can even actually *stretch* and *sigh* as you imagine and say to yourself or aloud, 'Oh, that feels *gooooood.. And smile a big stretchy smile.* Really get into it. What would you be thinking, how would your body feel? What emotions would you feel, happy, positive, optimistic, peaceful? *Keep doing this* until the alarm goes off. If you have time, repeat the visualisation in the evening.

Now, don't say you *can't*. Don't say you can't imagine what it would feel like to wake up from a great night's sleep. And *don't* say it makes you feel silly. This isn't going to feel right to start with. It might feel utterly alien and ridiculous, especially if you actually feel like death!

But you can start *somewhere*. And any feeling you can visualise that is better than where you are now, *is better than where you are now!*

Now, while it's good to do this in the morning, it's also fine to do it at any other time of day. Try to pick a time when you are not too stressed. Your mind will be less active and you'll feel less resistance from negative thoughts. Eventually, you'll get used to this new positive feeling and it will begin to grow. And when it gets easy to do the visualisation, where once it was hard, you *know* that exciting changes are taking place!

****

If you really want to make this more powerful, combine it with the Acting-As-If Exercise. Get up from your visualisation like a new person, an ex-insomniac. Get up from your visualisation and 'act as if' you had been a normal good sleeper for as long as you can remember.

This is a wonderful exercise as it prepares your mind to think that way in reality. Remember, the subconscious mind cannot tell the difference between imagination and reality. The reason it panics and stops you sleeping before events is because you have programmed it to react that way. So, by simply imagining a different future, you tell your brain to react according to this new, positive future.

In 'preparation' for an important event, you could do a daily six-minute visualisation of how you would like the day and night to go. Start by visualising how you will feel in the daytime before the event, how relaxed and happy you will feel, imagine into the evening with a happy expectation of sleep. Imagine going to bed, lying down and falling asleep quickly.

Then move to morning time when you will visualise getting up from a *delicious, delightful* sleep. Imagine attending your event happy, relaxed and refreshed.

And once again, don't worry if the first few attempts at either of these exercises become sabotaged by your mind. A little practice will make it easier and easier.

'I was doing really, really well. But now I have a hugely important event looming and I just don't feel I can cope. I'm thinking of cancelling and starting all this again when I'm feeling more confident. Is this a good idea?'

People often write and ask, 'Should I postpone my holiday?' or 'Should I cancel my 40th birthday party?' Or even 'Should I put off starting a family'!

If you are serious about reinventing yourself as a good sleeper, you must stop cancelling events and avoiding risks. Refusing to take tiny risks and thereby avoiding potentially stressful situations is one of the worst insomnia-reinforcing behaviours you can have.

By avoiding the event, you may avoid insomnia for one night, but at the same time, you reinforce insomnia as a life-long problem.

At the end of the day, you need to make the decision yourself of whether to attend a particular scary event and your decision will probably depend on where you consider yourself to be with your recovery. In the very early stages, big events could terrify you and sabotage your progress. But if you have already seen good improvement and are looking to take the leap towards Good Sleeper Identity, then you should be *planning* these events, not avoiding them.

Let's look at an example: suppose you have been invited to a big weekend away with friends and the thought of the effect on your sleep is already beginning to stress you out. The following are three possible outcomes to such an invitation. If you prefer, replace 'weekend away with friends' with your own personal anxiety-producing situation.

1. You decline the invitation, stay at home *and sleep fine.*

2. You say 'I might go', try to pretend the event isn't even happening, putting off your decision until the last minute, fuss and fret about how best to sleep that night, manage to 'fool yourself' *and you do sleep.*

3. You agree to go straight away, and look forward to the event *but do not sleep.*

Can you see that the *only* outcome which is in keeping with the identity of a really good sleeper is option 3, *even though you do not sleep?* Options 1 and 2, in which *you do sleep,* are examples of *insomnia-reinforcing behaviour.* According to options 1 and 2, you do manage to sleep, but at what future cost? By engaging in insomnia-reinforcing behaviour, you have ensured that next time you are put in this situation, you will suffer the same worry, the same anxiety, the same dilemma.

But in plumping for option 3, you take a risk and do not sleep. However, you have replaced unhelpful, reinforcing behaviour with normal behaviour. Even though you don't sleep *on this particular* occasion, this counts as a *successful step*. The old pattern has been weakened and you are one step further along the road to recovery. Keep this up, accept every invitation, look forward to having fun until *there will no longer be any safety to be found in saying no.* It won't be long before you will happily accept every invitation, look forward to every event *and sleep like a baby!*

Personally, this is how I dealt with these sorts of situation to eventually completely overcome my special event insomnia:

1. I would think to myself, 'I'm going away for the weekend (*Bring it on*), and I'm going to have a good time (*Expect the best*). I might sleep, I might not sleep, and I don't care either way' (*Let everything be okay*).

2. In the early days, I would use the six-minute visualisation once a day until the event and use the Stop Thinking Technique 'in the moment' whenever a fearful thought popped into my head. (Eventually, these techniques became unnecessary.)

3. I would go to bed at a normal time before the event, whenever I felt like it, with no special bedtime preparation or conditions *(acting like a normal good sleeper)*.

Did I sleep? Why bother asking? Whether I did or didn't actually sleep is irrelevant. My focus was on the event, not the sleep. It doesn't matter what happened – the outcome *was* okay.

As it happened, when I followed these steps, the outcome would usually be that I *would* sleep fine, even when there was still considerable fear left. When I didn't sleep, I paid as little attention to the lack of sleep as possible. Slowly, slowly, the association of special event and insomnia weakened and eventually vanished.

I think one of the main reasons that these sorts of events cause such a problem is just because they happen rarely. They pop up from time to time and this means it is very difficult to break this particular habit. After all, how can you create a habit for sleeping well before weddings, for example, when you may only be invited to half a dozen weddings in a lifetime? One future event can loom like a huge iceberg in the distance and cause you to worry about your sleep for weeks until there is little or no chance of your sleeping on the night before it.

If you really want to get over this most tenacious type of insomnia there is one sure way.

The best way out of this dreadful pattern is to give your system a short, sharp shock over a fortnight, or even a week. If you have some holiday time coming up, you could use it in the following way to get over your problem for good.

Make a plan to do something that would normally have affected your sleep *every single day*. Fill your days with activities that would normally have caused you some anxiety about sleeping. When you have something to look forward to *every* day, fun events assume less significance. Try to plan at least one thing to do every day and make sure some of these things involve an early start. This will get you used to the feeling of planning, of looking forward, of having fun and enjoying your life again. This can be hard if you have no holiday time free, work long hours and have little money, but if you can arrange it, a week or two like this could change your life.

What a fantastic way to begin your reinvention as a good sleeper. And when the time is over, continue to find something, however small, to look forward to about every tomorrow.

I still remember the first time I arranged a whole weekend's activities for myself and my friends. A few years previously I wouldn't even have had enough friends to do this, let alone have the confidence to organise an whole weekend for them. At night I relaxed into to my safety thought – 'I've done it before, I can do it again.'

I slept fine the whole weekend and during the day I was having too good a time to worry or care about how I was sleeping! I celebrated this weekend for weeks. I thought about the occasion whenever I could, and smiled at the memory. I now had a massive, strong safety net, and it was growing! It felt amazing, like my life was starting!

Seek out special events, plan special events, *look forward* to special events. Act as normally as you can … and then be okay with the outcome, no matter what happens. Do this enough times, and the old habit *will* break down. Keep avoiding special events, and the old insomnia habit *will* continue.

You Cannot Let It Slip

This dream of every chronic insomniac is to move beyond insomniac, to become, not a recovering insomniac, but an *ex-insomniac*. You want sleep to be effortless, automatic, inevitable, the furthest thing from your mind.

In a sense, reinventing yourself as a good sleeper is a leap of faith. And just as with any leap of faith, there can be no faltering, no turning back. You must at some point decide that the reinvention is now complete. You now expect the best, you always let everything be okay, and you no longer make compromises to your life for the sake of sleep, *ever*. You must decide to act and speak as a good speaker, *always*. You are no longer picking scary things off a list; you are now living exactly the life you would as if you were a normal good sleeper. If you go through a normal bad patch of sleep, you may want to tighten up on sleep hygiene for a bit. Other than that, there should be no more special consideration. There is *no* more compromise, none whatsoever. There is no more reading, no researching, no sleep therapy. There are no special considerations, there is no more hesitating about whether to do something you really want to do.

If you falter and fuss and wonder about whether this is a good idea, and worry about whether you are doing it right, then you could just end up confused, frustrated and lose trust in the process. So only take the step once you are completely confident that you can follow through. Once you take the step, you need to live your life from this point on according to this new identity, *always*.

So don't write and tell me you tried this and it didn't work. Those people who have moved to this stage do not contact me. They do not complain that it isn't working. This is only to be attempted once you are willing no longer to entertain thoughts of it 'working' or not. They do not scrutinise the instructions to make sure they are getting them right. They may not even own my book any more.

But, at some point, this change needs to happen. At some point you need to start thinking, acting, living your life from the place of a great sleeper.

When you feel the reinvention process is nearing completion, take this book to the charity shop or pass it on to someone else who needs it. Don't buy any more sleep books I may write. Unsubscribe from my emails. After all, why would a normal good sleeper subscribe to an insomnia mailing list? Forget about sleep, forget about insomnia, forget about this book, throw away the ladder, *and get on with your life.*

The Good Sleeper Club Rules:
(And These *Are* Rules)

1. *Expect the best*, assume that your sleep will become brilliant, perfect.

2. *Let everything be okay* – never, ever negatively judge your sleep. See only good, and deny all that could be judged as bad.

3. *Bring it on* – get on with your life without one single compromise to your sleep.

ॐ

Conclusion
It only works if you do it
The inevitable section for tough nuts

'There are thousands of books on positive thinking out there.
If it were this easy, we'd all be doing it.
Why can't you just tell me how to sleep?'

You're right. There *are* a lot of books out there. But did you know that only a small proportion of people ever finish reading a book, and a much, *much* smaller number ever follow the instructions in any book?

I think a lot of people genuinely believe that they can read a book and by some sort of osmosis, this will cause them to overcome chronic insomnia. Many people, used to a quick-fix with sleeping pills, imagine that an insomnia book is some literary equivalent of a sleeping pill. 'Oh yes, I really want to get over this!' they claim. But they don't want to have to actually do anything.

'I hate to admit it, but I'm reluctant to start the programme. I just
have a nagging feeling this won't work for me.
And if I don't believe it will work, it won't.'

If you went to the doctor with a headache, and the doctor gave you pills, you may or may not take them. But you wouldn't go back to the doctor and say, 'Doctor, I didn't take those pills you gave me and they're not working.' So don't give me excuses and arguments. Don't tell me you can't or won't do this, that or the other. Don't tell me you can't think positively. Don't tell me you are a scientist and don't believe in positive thinking. And *don't* write and tell me all the reasons you didn't follow the instructions and in the same breath tell me this method doesn't work.

Are you waiting for someone to 'fix' you? Are you are waiting for me to 'do' something to you, to take away your insomnia? If so, you will have a long wait. No one is going to be able to put this right for you. No one will 'cure' you. No one will ever 'fix' you. All that I, or any therapist, can do, is to show you the way. You are going to have to take the steps, the actions yourself. Be one of those who take control of their own lives.

Following the Method means following the Method. It does not mean picking and choosing. It does *not* mean reading the book, getting all psyched up and positive, and thinking that's going to do it.

> The true value to an individual of any new strategy or skill
> is in direct proportion to the frequency of its use
>
> (Anthony Robbins)

Don't imagine you can just read a book and your life will miraculously get better. You can't just read it; you have to *do* it, *all* of it. And that includes:

1. doing your very best to be positive even when, no, *especially when*, you haven't slept well, and

2. giving it time. When I say this takes time, *I mean that this TAKES TIME.* Doing it (properly) includes giving it

enough time for the promises to start really affecting your beliefs, and this may well be a couple of months or longer.

Sometimes people write to me after just a few days and say, 'I started your Method three days ago and it's not working. I'm giving up.' (Just for the record, following the Method does *not* include complaining after three days.)

I didn't get to perfect sleep overnight. I didn't get here through fussing and falling to bits whenever it went wrong. I didn't get here through sending a barrage of emails to therapists with dozens of precisely detailed questions (although I had previously done just that for many years). In the end, I *had* no one else to ask. It was all down to me; me and my thoughts. And *that* is how you need to view this. You need to start looking within, watching your own thinking, and taking control of it.

Don't write to tell me you can't, or that this doesn't work, or that you tried but you couldn't keep it up. *I can't do this for you. NO ONE can do this for you.* So please don't think up excuses for why you can't do the techniques. Don't let the internal saboteur stop you from continuing with the positive thinking.

Are you someone who reads *about* insomnia? Are you someone who always has their own personal reasons for not following instructions, and for not doing techniques? Did you read my first book and angrily reject it because you didn't find the answer you were looking for? Did I not give you *the* answer? You won't find the answer in this book. The answer is not to be found in reading the advice, but in *following* the advice. The answer is not intellectual, it is experiential.

I once knew a chap who had aspirations of becoming a Buddhist, of finding 'enlightenment'. He was also a deep thinker and a great intellectual. But because he was such an intellectual, he spent all his spare time just reading books about Buddhism. I suggested many times that he should attempt to meditate, because according to the books, meditation was the way to happiness, peace and enlightenment. But while he would read and read *about* meditation, he almost never meditated in all the years I knew him. He was still seeking for *understanding*, for the *answer to all his questions.* He was seeking peace through reading *about* peace, trying to *understand* peace, testing theories *about* peace. And, at least while I knew him, he never found enlightenment or any peace of mind and continued to be one of the most anxious and unhappy people I have ever known. Don't be like my Buddhist friend.

In the very first chapter of this book I said my intention was to switch on the light in your brain; that the only way to overcome your problem was to bring you to an understanding of your own problem and the way this works for you. But this type of understanding is no good if it remains a mere idea in your mind. It is of no use if all that understanding disappears the moment you suffer a setback. You need to bring that understanding into your experience, into your life. *You need to live it.*

You need to *feel and believe* you are getting better during a really good stretch of sleep.

You need to *experience* a really bad night, and still have a really good, productive day.

You need to *notice* that your negative thinking lessens when you simply make a small effort to change your thoughts.

You need to experience, feel, believe (not just read) that by doing all these seemingly ineffectual things I suggest, *your problem starts to lessen, your thinking becomes more positive, and your sleeping gets better!*

'But when I do all this positive thinking,
sometimes I feel like I'm telling lies.'

So tell lies. No, I mean it. Tell lies about your sleep. Fake it, for as long as it takes for your mind to start believing it (at which point it becomes a lie no longer). The fact that you don't believe the affirmations yet is exactly as it should be. The fact that visualisation is hard and feels wrong is *exactly* as it should be! The fact that stopping thinking feels difficult is exactly as it should be! We are looking for a *new* belief, not an old one. That means a *new* repeated thought, *not* an old one! And of course a new thought is going to feel strange, different, silly or untrue at first. The idea is to start thinking the new positive thought as often as you can, until it stops sounding wrong, starts to 'stick', and you begin to really believe it. Belief change *can* happen through external circumstances (such as actually sleeping better) but it can also be affected directly, by actively repeating a new thought as often as you possibly can. Eventually, this has to have the effect of changing your belief. It is just how the human mind works.

Choose what you would like to be true, and tell that story from now on.

'But I am a very anxious person naturally and I have a lot of
other issues besides insomnia. I just don't believe this will work
for someone with as many problems as I have.'

Do I sound sane to you? Do I sound like a paragon of British composure? Believe me, it wasn't always this way. While I may sound completely stable and sorted, once upon a time, this was really not the case. I have a massively overactive mind, a leaning towards neuroses, OCD and a tendency to bouts of depression. If I had had the slightest shred of faith in the ability of doctors to help with depression and mental illness, no doubt I would have been diagnosed with all sorts of disorders. I would probably have been on bucket-loads of pills. I never seriously considered suicide but sometimes I really did empathise with those who took that route. I honestly considered looking for a heroin dealer because I heard that heroin gives the most amazing, ecstatic sleep. Luckily, I don't move in the sorts of circles where I could find such stuff. Who knows where I would have ended up if I had managed to get hold of hard drugs? I worked myself into a total panic many, many times. Just hearing or reading the word 'sleep' would bring on an attack of palpitations. My tummy would 'flip' a hundred times a day and whenever I remembered my terrible problem. I remember often driving out into the countryside so I could scream. I became so anxious at a party once I collapsed with a violent vomiting attack. I would burst into tears in the street. And I often would engage in the classic crazy behaviour – sitting on the edge of my bed, just rocking, rocking, rocking.

I was a total nutcase.

And now ... I sleep better than anyone I know, and life is good. I'm still a bit nuts. I'm still obsessive, a little neurotic. But these days I like to think that just adds to my creativity and is all part of my charm.

So please don't think you are too unstable, too anxious, too crazy to take control of your thinking and overcome your insomnia. I can out-crazy the lot of you.

Many self-help books are written by seemingly perfect people. People who are unflappable, profoundly non-judgemental, living in the moment and at peace with themselves and the world. They may take on a semi-religious tone and appear as some kind of spiritual guru, even a God substitute.

You will be reassured to know that I am none of these things. I eat too much, probably drink a bit too much. I'm disorganised, untidy, moody, often irrational and I don't read *The Guardian* or campaign against slavery.

But *I sleep*. You do not need to be a perfect human being in order to sleep. You do not need to become a model of self-help perfection. You do not need to find enlightenment. You can be *you*, with all your wonderful flaws and imperfections, *and still sleep like a baby*.

These days, when I want to change something, I don't do anything practical such as sitting down and making plans, or getting advice or therapy[4] – I just start telling a new story. It may be all nonsense to begin with, but pretty soon I start believing ... and *then* the story tends to come true. (I'm a big believer in 'faking it 'til you make it'.)

'But after all I've been through, can I ever really become a great sleeper?'

Yes, you can. But I cannot tell you how long it will take before you get there. The speed at which you make a total recovery will largely be down to *choice*.

When you finally decide to say to yourself, 'I will take whatever comes my way, be it sleep, or lack of it', then you have made that

---

[4] I'm not suggesting you don't go and get professional help for emotional issues or mental illness. But don't let the presence of other emotional problems lead you to reject the suggestions in this book for dealing with your insomnia. Let my advice *complement* your medical treatment.

choice. When you can do this, it doesn't really ever come back; at least, not in its previous virulent form.

Let me assure you, if you have *any* experience of sleeping better due to 'positive thinking', or of changing your thoughts and seeing a positive result in your sleep, *then you can become a brilliant, natural, effortless sleeper.* That same mechanism that allowed thought to keep you awake on one single night can be reversed. Then, it can be strengthened and honed to making you into the world's greatest sleeper.

I believe this is true because I am now becoming a greater and greater sleeper all the time. I … who was once convinced I had an incurable physical disease, who thought I was broken, different, for whom nothing ever worked. Who had aches, pains, 'heart jumps', tummy flips, rushes of adrenaline, moments of terror and panic, days and nights of desolate misery in a pit of black despair …

I have been where you are now, or worse. And it was by following this same advice that I now sleep better than almost everyone I know.

I got to this happy place through a constant but fairly *slow* improvement. Once I had made the initial breakthrough, I simply focused on the good and completely ignored the bad. I did keep my sleep hygiene tight for the first few months but other than that, I put my life first and tried to live as much like a normal sleeper as I could. *That was basically it.* I paid no attention to the specific aspects of my remaining problem. I did a lot of pretending, a lot of faking, a lot of jollying myself up, until I didn't need to fake it any more. It had become my reality.

'So chronic insomnia really can be cured?'

Absolutely, it can.

You know, it has often crossed my mind that I could actually quite easily have a 'relapse' (my most hated word!) I could *very easily* go back to being a really terrible sleeper, completely obsessed with my problem again, trying one pill after another. I could spend the next 30 or 40 years as a chronic insomniac.

How?

If I focused on the bad nights (which still very occasionally happen), the way I am feeling moment to moment, on every strange flutter, twitch or 'funny feeling', on the possibility that this, that or the other will affect my sleep, if I went back to researching, reading, talking about insomnia. If I *stopped* talking about how great my sleep is, if I looked to the negative instead of always, *always* to the positive, *I could go back there too!*

Instead, I pay no attention whatsoever to a less than perfect night, I don't give more than a second to a negative thought. I simply won't allow a negative sleep thought any space in my head. If one pops in, I just think *negative thought – be gone!* And change my mind to a more worthwhile subject. I don't even keep up to date with current research about sleep, although I am under great pressure to do so. People send me links, text me about TV programmes: 'You must watch this documentary about sleep!' they say. But I never watch them. I live the life of a great sleeper, always. I maintain this identity always, even in the face of apparent threats to it.

And do you know? It's *this commitment* that's keeping me away from the most monumental relapse! It's all that's keeping me from a 30-year problem. Seriously!

But, don't be alarmed. Most of what's keeping you from being where I am now is cultivating the same way of thinking. You can just as easily join me in this happy place. You can become one of the Good Sleepers, one of the *Great* Sleepers. Take back your control, of your mind, your sleep and your life. You are far more powerful and able to do this than you realise.

Do you know how I can *know* that insomnia will never come back for me? It's because I no longer care whether or not I will sleep. If I miss a night, I pay no attention to it. If I missed two, three nights, because of circumstances beyond my control, I wouldn't be happy about it, but it wouldn't signal insomnia for me. I wouldn't panic. I would just get on with life and look forward to sleeping again. The difference between a few bad nights and 'insomnia' is the label you give.

When the bad times hit, please resist the temptation to give up and start something else, because this stuff works. But it doesn't work like clockwork. It doesn't work according to hard and fast laws. Sometimes bad nights and bad stretches come along for no reason whatsoever. It is at these times that you really must keep the faith, know that what you are doing is right, refocus and sit it out, waiting for things to pick up again. They always do.

You know all those little clichés, *Life is what you make it; you create your own reality; if you keep doing what you're doing, you'll keep getting what you're getting; if you want to change your world, change your thoughts … ?*

It turns out they are all true.

But for our purposes there is really only one you need to remember. I leave you with one last saying, my favourite one of all.

The story you tell about your sleep will come true.

CPSIA information can be obtained at www.ICGtesting.com
Printed in the USA
LVOW10s1614040115

421453LV00021B/566/P